I Woke Up One Day and I Was 40

I Woke Up One Day and I Was 40

◆

A Man's Guide to Fitness and Health...
Just 29 Days to Changing Your Life

Tony Vercillo

iUniverse, Inc.
New York Lincoln Shanghai

I Woke Up One Day and I Was 40
A Man's Guide to Fitness and Health...Just 29 Days to Changing Your Life

iUniverse books may be ordered through booksellers or by contacting:

iUniverse
2021 Pine Lake Road, Suite 100
Lincoln, NE 68512
www.iuniverse.com
1-800-Authors (1-800-288-4677)

ISBN: 0-595-33910-7 (pbk)
ISBN: 0-595-67032-6 (cloth)

Printed in the United States of America

Contents

Part III   *Get Ready...Set...Action!*

Acknowledgements

There are many people I'd like to thank. First, my entire family, for putting up with all my crazy ideas. Second, my children, Anthony, Darien, and Nicolas, for allowing Dad to fulfill his dreams while occasionally missing that important soccer, basketball, or hockey game; and thanks to Donna Peerce, for providing structure, editing, and her keen writing insight. Finally, thanks to my chiropractor, golf partner, and best friend, Dave Martin, for keeping me "straight."

Preface

✦

The Wake-Up Call

o o o o o o o o o o o o o o o o o o o o o o o o o o o o o o o o o o o
"To me, old age is always fifteen years older than I am."
—*Bernard Baruch on his 85th birthday, August 20, 1955*

It was still dark when I woke up. I turned over on my other side and snuggled back under the covers, trying to go back to sleep. I couldn't. All was quiet in the house yet there I was restless and wide-awake. I looked over at the clock on the bedside table and saw that it was only 3:00 a.m. *Why was I waking up so early?* Ah yes…I remembered. It was my 40th birthday, July 3rd. I threw back the bedcovers and sat on the side of the bed, feeling as if a boulder had just rolled over me, waking me, shaking me…making me stare hard at my life and my priorities. I gazed out the window where a streetlight shone brightly. I couldn't believe it. I was 40 years old. Life was passing me by. *40? When did that happen? Was my life half over?* Mortality stood above me like the grim reaper; staring me in the face, letting me know who I was, where I was in life, and the nature of my existence. *I was getting old.* Reality, along with Mortality, hit me like a ton of bricks. I was 40 years old and it was time to grow up.

I had always been very athletic as a young adult and even boxed for 5 years. While growing up, I was involved in martial arts and sports. I had dreams of becoming a star basketball player in the NBA, or maybe a race car driver, or even a middleweight boxing champion. But, there I was—40 years old—and I was none of those things. I knew that I had to face reality and accept the fact that I'd never be any of those things I dreamed about in my early adulthood.

Was this the end? Was it over for me?

Don't get me wrong. My life was good. *Exceptionally* good. I was doing what I love to do. I lived in one of the most exclusive, richest areas in Los Angeles and drove a Jaguar. I was—by LA's standards—on top of the world—a successful entrepreneur and businessman.

On the surface, my life looked golden. But, I didn't *feel* golden. I was stressed and burned out. For many years, I had been working long hours and slaving away 7 days a week to obtain all the riches and material possessions that money could buy. I was driven to be wealthy.

I'm not sure why I was so driven. Maybe it was because I grew up in Brooklyn—one of 6 children in a working middle-class family. Maybe it was because we didn't have much in the way of material things and after I grew up, I wanted more. Maybe I just wanted my Dad to be proud of me…I don't know. Maybe it was all these things and more that made me become a slave to money.

I remembered my father on his deathbed, when he took my hand and looked me straight in the eyes and said, "Tony, one day you're gonna wake up and realize that money isn't important—that family, children, and building the next generation is your true legacy." I remember looking at my father and saying, "Yea, yea…." Just to appease him, of course. But, I hadn't really listened. I was too caught up in my super fast, *rich* lifestyle to really listen. I didn't want to listen.

However, at that bleak moment, when I turned 40, and while the world was still asleep and quiet, I wondered what kind of legacy I'd leave in life. *That I owned an expensive sports car and lived in a million dollar home?* Is this what my children would talk about when they discussed their father? I had fallen into the trap—thinking that success was based on how large my house was and the type of car I drove. More specifically, I had fallen into the *Los Angeles* society trap and my priorities were all out of whack.

While sitting on that bed, I looked at my body—gave it a hard look. I was 6 ft. tall with brown hair and eyes. Fairly attractive. Typical Italian-looking type of guy. My stomach was beginning to protrude and I knew I wasn't as physically in shape as I could be, although I had been working out diligently since my mid 30s. With the out-of-shape body that I had, along with the long hours of working, how long would I live? I could hear my son saying, *"Yea, my Dad worked so hard, he had a heart attack at a young age…but, we were rich."* I didn't want to leave that kind of legacy for my children. Surely, there was more to my life than that.

Truth was, I didn't feel very healthy. I had been living in the fast lane for so long—trying my best to keep up with and *surpass* the Jones's, that I had forgotten what it was like to just stop and contemplate about where I was headed. I was also very upset that I hadn't achieved *more* in my life. It always seemed like I should be doing more. I should have become a famous racecar driver or middleweight boxing champion. *Would that have made my Dad proud?* I found myself wallowing in misery that I, Tony Vercillo—at 40—could no longer be any of those things. I realized that I was simply a washed-up *'thousandnaire'* who was burning out fast. To make matters worse, my cholesterol level was off the charts!

Then, it hit me. An *awakening*. An *epiphany*. Sitting there on my bed on that warm July morning, with the moon still glowing high in the sky, it hit me. I could take charge of my life and become better. I could rearrange my priorities and start enjoying life the way my father always preached. I could become the best that I could be at 40 and beyond. That it's not the end, but rather, the beginning of a new way of life.

I realize there are many men out there who are turning 40, 50, 60 or beyond. And all of you might be experiencing the same reality check that I experienced on my 40th birthday. Trust me, it's not too late to change your life and become the best you can be. It's not too late to lose weight, become strong and fit, and to align your priorities in a way that supports optimum health and happiness.

It doesn't matter if you make a million dollars. It doesn't matter if you become that famous racecar driver or the next Muhammad Ali. It doesn't matter if you live in a multi-million dollar home or drive a Jaguar. None of those things matter. What does matter is optimum health, family, friends, and love. If you have love and good health, then you have everything. That's all there is. And, if you have physical health and vitality, chances are the other things in your life will fall in place—love, family, and friends. There's something magical about being healthy and the owner of your life—your destiny. It makes you more confident in every other area and as a result, improves your relationships with family and friends.

Because of that early morning "wake-up" call, I decided to write a book to help all of you men out there who are turning 40 or beyond. This book is different than the other fitness books you'll find out there on the market. Many books address fitness and health for young men, but there are very little that focus on men who are 40 and beyond. And we might just be the ones who need it most!

In addition, this book is different because I'm *not* your typical diet guru or so-called fitness expert. I've never been on "Oprah" or "Dateline" with my "expert" advice (although I might be after this book!) I've never been quoted in *Health & Fitness Magazines*. But, what's *more important* is that I think you will relate to me because I'm a regular guy just like you. Sure, maybe I earned more money at one time or maybe *you* earned more than I did! But, we're all just regular guys in this world who are trying to make a living and provide for our families and loved ones. That makes all of us alike no matter what our financial status is.

I'm like you in the way that I like to golf, play basketball, watch movies, go out to dinner, watch my children in school activities and sports, and all those other things that regular people like to do. Perhaps I am only unique because I recognized at age 40 that I had to change my priorities or I might not be around to see my children grow up. That I might not be around to hold my grandbabies or coach Little League. I was fortunate to recognize this at the young age of 40. Many people don't recognize this until they're on their deathbed and even then, they might not get it. So, there I sat on my 40th birthday and I knew without a shadow of a doubt—I wanted to change my priorities and get my life in order—plus, get my body in top physical health.

When your body is in optimum condition, you will discover, as I have, that you will enjoy amazing energy, youth, and vitality—no matter what your age is. And, with that newfound energy, your possibilities are actually limitless. Not only will you feel great physically, but you will also have a mental clarity that will help you take control of your future and make your dreams a reality. Yes, *even at 40!*

I am now one of America's leading consultants, entrepreneurs, and health-care enthusiasts and for more than 20 years I've been sharing my secrets to success and good health with audiences around the world. Because of my wake-up call, I now want to share my tips and methods for changing an aging body into a youthful, strong, and very healthy body. I want to show you how to take care of your body and become the best that you can be. Let this book be your coach and your guide. It's not too late. Trust me. If I can do it, you can do it.

If you follow the tips and methods in this book, you can change your life in just 29 days. It has been said that it takes a month—29-30 days to create a habit—that if you do something over and over for a month, it will become a habit—something that you don't have to think about—you just do it. So, if you read this book and stick with me, then in just 29 days, you can change your life and be well on your way to a healthy, strong, fit body. Not only will you be on your way to a healthy body, but you'll also be on your way to improving your life in all areas—romance, relationships, finances, love. A healthy body will give you that amazing energy to improve all areas of your life and to ultimately achieve your dreams and happiness.

I invite you to join me on this journey—this adventure—to good health, good priorities, and a good youthful life. I guarantee you—it's not too late to become happy and fit.

Tony Vercillo

Getting Started

Before we get started, I wanted to give you an overview of what you need to do right now. This is a mini portion of my book. I am breaking with tradition by describing the art before I paint you the picture. These few tips will help you launch your new lifestyle and health plan.

The first thing I want you to do is estimate your daily caloric intake. Let's say it's 3,500 calories per day. This is now your baseline measure. As you eliminate foods or drink from your diet, you need to be sure you do not increase your caloric intake through other food groups. If you learn anything from this book, learn that losing weight is merely a mathematical formula. Eat 500 calories per day less than your norm and burn 500 calories per day with exercise and you will lose 2 pounds per week—period! Let's rock.

Week One

- Eliminate caloric drinks—worth approximately 120 calories per 12 oz. At 3 drinks per day, that's 360 calories each day and 2,520 calories per week that you've saved. This step alone will cause you to lose one pound every ten days. Replace caloric drinks with water or unsweetened (and decaf) ice tea.

- *Bonus Elimination: Stop drinking alcohol. If you must drink, go with one glass of wine per day as studies have shown that wine may be beneficial to your heart.*

- *Bonus Addition: Add a multi-vitamin with at least 500mg of C, and 50mg of each of the essential B vitamins. Your multi-vitamin should also include traces of magnesium, selenium, and zinc. If not, take an additional supplement that has at least the minimum daily requirement for each of these essential minerals.*

Week Two

- Eliminate all breads and potatoes (most starches). At three servings per day, these are estimated to be worth 400 calories/day and 2,800 weekly. By the end of week two, you will have reduced your caloric intake by 5,320 calories and you will lose approximately 1.5 pounds per week at this level.

- **Bonus Elimination:** *Stop drinking caffeinated drinks such as coffee, soft drinks, and even iced tea. Slowly wean yourself off the hard stuff and go to decaf. Convert to diet/caffeine free drinks.*

- **Bonus Addition:** *Add four 8 oz. glasses of water per day (on top of drinking other zero calorie liquids made primarily of water at each meal) and the supplements CoQ10, Omega 3, and Lipoeic Acid.*

Week Three

- Eliminate desserts and most sugars (zero calorie sweetener is O.K.). At 3 desserts per week, this is worth approximately 1,500 calories. Your cumulative total should now be 6,820 calories LESS than when you started. You will now lose close to 2 pounds per week.

- **Bonus Elimination:** *Stop smoking. Buy the 'patch' or another smoke-aid and finally kick this nasty habit.* Your wives, girlfriends and family will love you for this one!

- **Bonus Addition:** *Substitute 3 fruits in your diet for other food choices daily. Add a banana to your morning with non- or low-fat cereal. (Use low-fat or skim milk also). Have an apple at mid-morning, then perhaps an orange at mid-afternoon. Carry fruits with you to work. They're easy and inexpensive treats and your waistline will thank you!*

Week Four

- Convert to non-fat or low-fat milk, yogurt, and salad dressing. Every piece of food you eat at this point should be scrutinized for caloric and fat gram values. Opt for low-fat peanut butter, non-fat mayonnaise, low-fat cottage cheese, low-fat pasta sauce, etc. This should cut an additional 400 calories per day out of your diet, and 2,800 more by the end of the week. This now brings the total to 9,600 calories LESS than your baseline, which will enable you to lose around 2.5 pounds/week.

- **Bonus Elimination:** *Eliminate any/all unnecessary drugs, particularly those with ingredients that either cause your heart to race, or cause you to feel "loopy."*

- **Bonus Additions:** Add Lecithin (500mg), Calcium, and Glucosomine to your daily vitamin/mineral regimen. *And, get 8 hours of sleep per night, period. Be* *particularly sensitive to sleeping during the hours of 10 p.m. and 2 a.m., which is when your body regenerates most of its immune system.*

Day 29

- Pig Out! You deserve it. You've done a great job. That's right, have whatever you want on this day, then start the cycle all over again.

- Repeat the cycle on an ongoing basis and you will not only lose weight, but you will start to feel vibrant without all the ups and downs related to fatigue.

A Reminder

Stop for a moment and think about what these terrible vices are doing to your body. Consider the following examples:

Vice	Drug	Causes	What it does to your body
Smoking	Nicotine	Stimulant	Heart to race
Drinking	Alcohol	Depressant	Liver Damage
Drinking	Caffeine	Stimulant	Heart to race
Drugs	Marijuana	Depressant	Kills brain cells

Smoking

While smoking has long been linked to an array of health problems, recent research from the U.S. surgeon general found that smoking causes diseases in almost every organ of the human body. Released in late May of 2004, "The Health Consequences of Smoking: A Report of the Surgeon General," cites more than 1,600 scientific articles on the health effects of smoking. In addition to the well-known effects of smoking, such as lung, mouth and esophageal cancers, the new report found that smoking is conclusively linked to leukemia, cataracts and pneumonia as well as cancers of the pancreas, cervix and kidneys. Other complications linked to smoking in the report included diabetes complications, hip fractures and reproductive complications.

"The toxins from cigarette smoke can go everywhere the blood flows," said U.S. Surgeon General Richard Carmona, MD, MPH, FACS. "I'm hoping this new information will help motivate people to quit smoking and convince young people not to start in the first place."

Drinking Alcohol

There's probably nothing wrong with having a good ice cold beer on a hot summer afternoon, or a glass of Chardonnay with dinner. However, alcohol abuse is not a very healthy or attractive habit for anyone. People in their 40's who drink alcohol regularly could be increasing their risk of mild cognitive impairment, a precursor to dementia and Alzheimer's. The claim is reported in a 2004 issue of the *British Medical Journal.*

A number of factors determine the effect alcohol has on individuals—why different people consuming the same amount react differently or why the same person can have different reactions on different occasions.

- **Speed of Drinking:** The more rapidly the beverage is ingested, the higher the peak blood alcohol concentration (BAC). The liver metabolizes about 1/2 ounce of alcohol per hour.

- **Presence of Food in the Stomach**: Eating while drinking slows down the absorption rate. When alcoholic beverages are taken with a substantial meal, peak BAC may be reduced by as much as 50%.

- **Body Weight:** The larger person has more blood and requires greater amounts of alcohol to reach a given BAC.

- **Drinking History/Tolerance:** Increasing amounts of alcohol are needed to result in the physical and behavioral reactions formerly produced at lesser concentrations, if there is a long history of drinking.

- **Environment:** There may be differences in alcohol's effects, depending upon where one drinks (e.g., local bar, with family, hostile environment, etc.).

- **The Drinker's Expectations:** Many people become intoxicated on less alcohol merely because they have that expectation before they begin drinking.

- **General State of Emotional and Physical Health:** Many people seem more susceptible to the effects of alcohol when they are extremely fatigued, have recently been ill, or are under emotional stress and strain. The usual amount of alcohol may result in uncomfortable effects.

- **Sex Differences:** Given the same amount of alcohol and proportional body weight, females will generally have a higher BAC than their male counterparts.

- Females are generally more affected by alcohol just prior to menstruation.

- Females taking birth control pills or medications containing estrogen may remain intoxicated longer than those who do not, due to the liver's function of metabolizing both.

- **Other Drugs:** Prescription, over-the-counter, illicit and unrecognized drugs all have potential reactions with alcohol. One should be aware of the additive and synergistic effects when these drugs are mixed with alcohol.

Ill Effects of Smoking & Drinking Combined

Everyone has heard about the ill effects of smoking, but there's research that now proves smoking and drinking alcohol may affect the quality of your semen. *Ouch!* Not what we virile men want to hear!

A group of investigators from Argentina found that men who both drank alcohol and smoked cigarettes were more likely to have a smaller amount of semen, a lower concentration of sperm, and a lower percentage of active sperm than abstainers. However, these semen alterations were present only in men who both smoked and drank, and not in men with one habit but not the other.

For a normally fertile man, the reductions in semen quality are not enough to render him infertile, study author Dr. Marta Fiol de Cuneo told Reuters Health. However, in men who already have fertility problems, these sperm changes might make the situation worse, she said. "In conjunction with another deleterious factor they would diminish male fertility," said the researcher, who is based at the Universidad Nacional de Cordoba.

Cuneo explained that smoking and drinking together may exert "additive" or "synergistic" effects. In the case of synergy, this would mean that one factor enhances the effects of the other, she explained.

In the *Fertility and Sterility Journal,* she and her colleagues wrote that previous research had investigated the effects of either smoking or drinking on semen quality, with mixed results. However, many of those studies looked at only a small group of men, involved men who may have infertility problems, or could not separate the effects of smoking from drinking, since those habits often go hand in hand.

To investigate the question further, Cuneo and her colleagues asked almost 4,000 men between the ages of 29 and 36 about their smoking and drinking habits, and tested their semen. The researchers found that men who both smoked and drank showed changes in semen quality, which were not seen in men who had neither or either of these habits.

Men who drank less than 500 milliliters of wine per day—roughly equivalent to 3 glasses—had the same risk of semen changes as men who drank more, and men who limited their cigarettes to less than 20 per day showed similar risks to heavier smokers.

"Men who wish to procreate should be specifically warned of this matter," Cuneo and her colleagues stated.

So, guys, this study is one more example of why it's a good idea to stop smoking!

Marijuana & The Effects on the Brain

Scientists have learned a great deal about how marijuana acts in the brain to produce its many effects. When someone smokes marijuana, THC rapidly passes from the lungs into the bloodstream, which carries the chemical to organs throughout the body, including the brain.

In the brain, THC connects to specific sites called cannabinoid receptors on nerve cells and influences the activity of those cells. Some brain areas have many cannabinoid receptors; others have few or none. Many cannabinoid receptors are found in the parts of the brain that influence pleasure, memory, thought, concentration, sensory and time perception, and coordinated movement.

The short-term effects of marijuana can include problems with memory and learning; distorted perception; difficulty in thinking and problem-solving; loss of coordination; and increased heart rate. Research findings for long-term marijuana use indicate some changes in the brain similar to those seen after long-term use of other major drugs of abuse. For example, cannabinoid (THC or synthetic forms of THC) withdrawal in chronically exposed animals leads to an increase in the activation of the stress-response system and changes in the activity of nerve cells containing dopamine. Dopamine neurons are involved in the regulation of motivation and reward, and are directly or indirectly affected by all drugs of abuse.

One study has indicated that a user's risk of heart attack more than quadruples in the first hour after smoking marijuana. The researchers suggest that such an effect might occur from marijuana's effects on blood pressure and heart rate and reduced oxygen-carrying capacity of blood.

A study of 450 individuals found that people who smoke marijuana frequently but do not smoke tobacco have more health problems and miss more days of work than nonsmokers. Many of the extra sick days among the marijuana smokers in the study were for respiratory illnesses.

Even infrequent use can cause burning and stinging of the mouth and throat, often accompanied by a heavy cough. Someone who smokes marijuana regularly may have many of the same respiratory problems that tobacco smokers do, such as daily cough and phlegm production, more frequent acute chest illness, a heightened risk of lung infections, and a greater tendency to obstructed airways. Smoking marijuana increases the likelihood of developing cancer of the head or neck, and the more marijuana smoked the greater the increase. A study comparing 173 cancer patients and 176 healthy individuals produced strong evidence that marijuana smoking doubled or tripled the risk of these cancers.

40 and Beyond Fitness Tip:

Marijuana has the potential to promote cancer of the lungs and other parts of the body. Stay away from it!

Marijuana use also has the potential to promote cancer of the lungs and other parts of the respiratory tract because it contains irritants and carcinogens. In fact, marijuana smoke contains 50 to 70 percent more carcinogenic hydrocarbons than does tobacco smoke. It also produces high levels of an enzyme that converts certain hydrocarbons into their carcinogenic form—levels that may accelerate the changes that ultimately produce malignant cells. Marijuana users usually inhale more deeply and hold their breath longer than tobacco smokers do, which increases the lungs' exposure to carcinogenic smoke. These facts suggest that, puff for puff, smoking marijuana may increase the risk of cancer more than smoking tobacco.

No matter which way you look at it, guys, smoking marijuana is not a good choice.

I hope you've enjoyed this brief overview of some important facts regarding your health before you begin this book. Get ready for plenty more information as you are about to change your life and your health in a very positive way!

PART I

Checking in with Reality When You Hit 40

1

The Issue of Mortality

"We must be willing to get rid of the life we've planned, so as to have the life that is waiting for us."

—*Joseph Campbell*

Let's get one thing straight right now. Even though you're 40, you're not old. O.K.? Men (just like women) tend to think that once they hit 40, they're "over the hill," and life is about over for them. You may be embarking on a midlife crisis. In the next chapter, I'll discuss that more in-depth. For now, let's discuss mortality. Mortality strikes those who think they're "over the hill" like a brick, leaving them to feel that the next step is Rolaids, Tums, knee replacements, and *God forbid*, Pampers for Adults. (Do they even make those?) No wonder so many men hit a "middle-age" crisis during this time and start having affairs with young nubile women. It's in our genes to try to hold on to our youth. To buy toupees to cover those balding heads—to drive those Jags with the tops down on Sunset Boulevard and wink at the blondes driving by. We're all just trying to have a love affair with youth. That's all.

Sure, we human beings are mortal. We do have to die. It's a natural part of life—just the way birth is. But, we don't have to hasten our death with bad eating and exercising habits, or with bad attitudes. Plus, our spirits are immortal. Whatever we do in this life will live on and that part never dies. So, let's make our legacies rich and meaningful. Let's really make a difference in this world and in turn, every person and every tiny thing will be positively impacted.

Aha! I knew it. You think you're old at 40, don't you? I know I did. After all, the media and fitness magazines do everything they can to influence us to believe that only 20- and 30-year-olds are attractive and desirable, but that's not true. In fact, when you reach 40, you're just beginning to come into your own. You're just beginning to reach the point in life where you can be truly confident about who you are and where you stand in life measured against all those other men on the planet. It's a *good* thing. You've *earned* the right to be 40!

---

40 and Beyond Fitness Tip:

Take charge of your destiny.

Men in their 20s and 30s think they're invincible. I was one of them. We're the *Incredible Hulk* meets *Spiderman*. But, when you turn 40, you realize you can't do what you did in your 20s and 30s. All of a sudden, there are little aches and pains that scream out at you when you walk or get out of bed. All of a sudden, your clothes become tighter and you're buying the next size up. All of a sudden, you have a wife and children and there's the mortgage payment and you need a new car...and...STOP! Don't let the material things get the better of you.

Stop for just a moment and take a look at your mortality. Feel it. Know it. Embrace it. Then, look it in the eye and say, "Mortality, I'm not going to let you get the best of me today. I'm going to become stronger and healthier, so I'm in control—not you." Sure, it might feel a little silly talking to Mortality, but the fact is—we are all in charge of our destiny and the way we choose to spend our mortal life is up to us. If you want to run around in circles trying to keep up with the Jones's—all the while neglecting your body, your health, your family and loved ones, well, that's up to you. But, I think you're more like me. If you're reading this book, then you want to improve your life and become healthier. You want to re-prioritize your goals and really enjoy the best in life.

The First Excruciating Pain

I was only in my 30s when the *first* excruciating pain started. I was in Dallas, Texas, meeting a client over lunch. All of a sudden, sharp daggers of pain stabbed at my lower back. It was so intense, I fell out of my chair and rolled onto the floor like a withered up man in his 90s. Needless to say, after several guests in the restaurant ran over and helped me up, I was scared. I had no idea what was happening or if I was going to be crippled or have to live with this pain for the rest of my life.

I had to leave on the next plane that afternoon for home and took 4 Advil to help ease the pain, which radiated down my right leg and into my toes. The Advil barely touched the pain. I sat in First Class and again, doubled over in pain. If I tried to sit up, the pain was too excruciating—almost to the point of making me pass out.

The person sitting next to me recommended a chiropractor in Los Angeles and as soon as I could, I made an appointment. The chiropractor discovered that I had 2 compressed vertebrae at the bottom of my back. His prescription? To work out. To exercise and tone the body. "What?" I asked him. "Don't you want to give me a prescription for the pain? Some medicine that will help me?"

"Trust me," he said. "Exercise will do more good for you than all the medicine in the world. You're simply at that age where your muscles aren't as supple and flexible as they used to be."

"But, I don't have time to work out," I told him. "I run several businesses and work about 80 hours a week."

"That's another reason your back is so out of shape. The stress is killing you," he told me. "Everything works together—the mind and the body. You're not taking enough time to enjoy life. Working out will ease some of the stress and help you physically."

Unfortunately, as our age increases so does our risk for developing a lower-back problem. The American Academy of Orthopedic Surgeons reports that 80% of Americans will suffer some type of back pain in their lives. At this stage in your life it's very likely that you've already experienced some form of back pain like I did.

I listened to what the chiropractor told me and I began working out. I started playing more basketball and more golf. Anything active to increase my heart rate and tone my body. My chiropractor made me realize that I had to start focusing more on my health and physical fitness, or I would continue to have chronic pain. Later on in this book, I will highlight exercises and fitness tips to help you get in shape too.

Since then, this chiropractor and I have become the best of friends and together, we work out regularly every week. Gratefully, with his help, I started taking better care of my body when I was in my 30s, but it was only after I hit 40, that I began to focus on re-prioritizing my life in a more complete and comprehensive way, and as a result, improved my total state of being. If I hadn't met my chiropractor friend when I did, I'm not sure I'd even be here now to share this story with you. He may have saved my life.

As you age, several internal physiological changes have already begun. Hormone levels decrease, causing both sexual and psychological problems in men, and facilitating menopause and osteoporosis in women. Tendons weaken, collagen softens and joint surfaces wear, causing arthritis, tendonitis, and other aches and pains that annoy and ache at inopportune times. But, by eating right and getting the proper exercise, you can minimize all these things.

When we're in our 20s and 30s and are feeling strong and invincible, we often make bad choices and create bad habits. In fact, our bad choices can have alarming results. According to an article in *Psychology Today* in 1999, one-third of Americans are overweight, costing the U.S. government $100 billion each year in treatment of related illnesses. And since then, the rate has climbed even higher. In 1998, *Newsweek* reported that 65% of all Americans are overweight. Out of this, 80% of adults over the age 25 are overweight and one-quarter of those are clinically obese. What's even sadder is that juvenile obesity is also rising rapidly. In the United States, the incidence of obesity among children has more than doubled over the last 30 years.

> **40 and Beyond Fitness Tip:**
>
> *65% of all Americans are overweight and out of this, 80% of adults over the age of 25 are overweight and one-quarter of those are clinically obese.*

We go on diets, analyze and obsess about food, turn to it as an enemy or friend, eat too much, eat too little, worry about it, avoid it, crave it, revere it, or believe that a particular nutrient will magically melt the pounds. Yet despite all of our conscientious attention to food and the incredible advances we've made in nutritional science, not only are our waistlines continuing to increase, so, too, are most food-linked ailments. From high blood pressure, heart disease, and diabetes, to cancer, osteoarthritis, and depression, excess pounds are an ever-rising threat to our health and well-being. Americans continue to get fatter and fatter, and as they get fatter, mortality looms even closer. And, it's all because of bad choices. Choosing to live in the fast lane, not eating right, and not getting the proper exercise. It's like we look mortality in the eye and laugh at it, saying, "Hey! I'm young—I'm not going to die!"

It is important to understand mortality and to accept it. But, you just don't have to sit in that Lazy-Boy recliner in front of the television and wait for old age to overtake you. And, you don't have to run around in circles, slaving away to make that extra buck so you can have more than the Jones's. Because if that's all you do, then your bad choices will welcome old age and it will settle in…and fast!

40 and Beyond Fitness Tip:

Bad choices revolve around immediate rewards and we don't think about the price we'll pay later...So, instead focus on long-term healthy rewards and results.

Most of our bad choices in life revolve around an immediate reward. When we're in our 20s and 30s, we might be able to get away with drinking, smoking, roasting our skin in the hot sun, not exercising, and eating too much. The immediate rewards are seductive and *oh, so good!* And because of this, we choose to live in the moment and not think about the consequences—the fact that we'll pay the price later. When I had my back pain in my 30s, it was due to the fact that I hadn't taken time to exercise and keep my body limber. I ignored the fact that I needed to stop working so much and slow down. I was too caught up in making money and living in the fast lane. Because it felt good. It was exhilarating to be rich and be able to buy anything I wanted. But, I focused so much on material possessions, I lost track of who I was and where I was headed. I lost track of the things in life that are the most precious—family, friends, optimum health, and love. And, it caught up with me—early. It was easier to live in the moment and just *go, go, go,* and not think of what would happen if I didn't stop. That's so typical of feeling invincible when you're in your 20s and 30s.

Our desire to take the path of least resistance is so strong that we continue our sometimes destructive behavior—like smoking, overeating, laying out in the sun, and not exercising—even though we know it may literally kill us someday. We don't need to be slaves to instant gratification.

40 and Beyond Fitness Tip:

"I hated every minute of training, but I said, don't quit. Suffer now and live the rest of your life a champion."

Muhammad Ali

The key to breaking a bad habit and adopting a good one is making changes in our daily life that will minimize the influence of the *now* and remind us of the *later.* It sounds difficult, but it can be done. If you follow the tips and exercises in this book, then you'll be making changes in your daily life that will provide a positive impact on you for a lifetime.

When breaking a bad habit, you need to remember:

1. Minimize or avoid the immediate reward.

2. Make the long-term negative consequence seem even more immediate and important.

In other words, just imagine what your life is going to be like if you don't start living more healthfully. Imagine yourself bent over on an airplane the way I was, not able to stop the excruciating pain. Imagine not being able to walk up a flight of stairs because you're winded from smoking too much. Imagine not being able to play softball with your children because you get too tired and winded. These are just little things, but if you stop and think about it, you'll understand that you are mortal and you won't live forever…so, don't *help* mortality by continuing your bad habits.

---

40 and Beyond Fitness Tip:

"It is in the knowledge of the genuine conditions of our lives that we must draw our strength to live and our reasons for living."

Simone De Beauvoir

Most likely, it's going to be tough to break your bad habits and start good ones. But the potential long-term benefits are well worth it. I'm a living example of this.

It's never easy to change, but for some people, it is exceptionally difficult. Take baby steps and visualize the long-term rewards. Stick with me and continue to read this book, because I'll guide you and help you achieve the rewards you deserve. I'll help you remain young—yes, *even* at 40 and beyond!

Dreams

Some people who reach 40 just accept their mortality and give up on their dreams. When we're in our 20s and 30s, we feel quite immortal. But, now after 40…well, many people feel like they're too old to try to accomplish anything else in life. *Wrong!*

Use your dreams to make your life better and don't wait for *next year* to try to achieve those dreams. Everyone has dreams. Everyone has passions. Everyone has hopes. Neale Donald Walsch, author of *Conversations with God,* said, "Somewhere between 40 and 60 you've given up on your grandest dream, set aside your highest hope, and settled for your lowest expectation—or nothing at all."

---

40 and Beyond Fitness Tip:

It is important that you continue to dream and make plans to achieve those dreams.

This sums up the human experience perfectly through the process of neglect, ambivalence, and/or self-doubt. What could have been a life of enlightenment, creation, and achievement ends up as a life of utter disappointment and regret for most people. Don't let it. You can still achieve your dreams and reach for the highest star. It's not too late. You're not too old! Please, don't let fear hold you back.

Being Afraid of Fear

I hope I haven't scared you because I know that fear is a major factor in all our lives—in everything we do. And when we hit 40, sometimes fear might grab us and say, "Hey, you're too old to accomplish much of anything now." Could be that fear is stopping *you* from moving forward. Some people are afraid to change. It's true. And, even the word, *fear,* sounds scary itself. We're afraid of fear. In fact, fear can escalate into terror and terror can turn into frantic action or paralyzing inertia. And then, what happens? We stay in our trap of "aging." We think it's too late to change…too late to become better. Fear and Mortality work hand-in-hand to make us sit back and accept our situation and station in life.

---

40 and Beyond Fitness Tip:

Fear can be both positive and useful to help you change your attitude.

Because so many of our experiences with fear throughout life have been negative, we fail to see the positive and useful sides of fear. Fear can be both positive and useful. *What? Are you crazy?* you're saying right now. Let me explain. Fear says things like, "I'm afraid it's too late for me. I'm afraid my body is too far gone—that I'm too old—that I can't change my attitude…that I'll never be anything more than I am right now."

Fear alerts us to the things that need changing. It says, "Stop a moment and check this out." It is something that almost slips into our consciousness without us realizing it's there because fear has been around us all our lives. We barely notice when it's taking hold.

Fear can be a feeling—a "perception" that lets us know we have neglected something in our lives—that we need to stop and focus on it. That's what happened to me when I turned 40. I woke up early that morning, not able to sleep because something scared me. Mortality and fear took me by the arms and said, "We're here. Look at us." I was forced to re-examine my life and it didn't look good. I was scared. I was stressed out. That fear made me take charge of my destiny and embrace my humanity.

So, you can use fear in a positive way. If you're afraid of getting old—of dying—of not achieving those dreams of being healthy, fit and happy—then use that fear to do something about it. Notice the fear. Acknowledge it—just the way you acknowledge your mortality—and move onward.

Fear and Your Health

A recent article from *AM News* (a publication of the American Medical Association) addresses gender-specific attitudes toward healthcare. Men go to the doctor for issues relating to physical or sexual prowess, which doctors often view as lead-ins to discussing other topics. Hopefully, the recent advertising campaigns using sports figures such as Magic Johnson and Lance Armstrong talking about their own health issues (AIDS and cancer) will begin to change men's attitudes in this area.

It was reported in *Today's Health & Wellness Magazine*, that a 17-year-old male who died days after being treated for minor injuries received in a car accident, actually died from something that had not been known to the doctors. His death was initially blamed on internal injuries that were not immediately apparent, but an autopsy revealed that the young man had died of a blood clot in his lung caused by undiagnosed testicular cancer that had spread throughout his body. It was not a hidden cancer; the patient could not have been unaware of the five-inch mass on his testicle. Still, he had not sought medical care.

On average, women live six years longer than men do. Many believe that at least part of this phenomenon can be attributed to a lack of access to care, either because of men's fears or because of systemic issues such as a lack of insurance. Don't let this be you. If you have any unusual symptoms in your body, seek medical care. Do not let fear stand in your way of becoming a healthy, fit individual.

We must take personal responsibility for our fears and respond to them constructively. This means refusing to take on someone else's fear or project our fears onto others. It also means taking responsibility for our health by acting as our own healthcare team leader, talking openly with friends, family and healthcare practitioners and doctors, and expecting them to respond to us as the whole individuals we are. We must also pay as much attention to our dreams, intuition and knowledge as we do to logic, statistics, lab tests and usual and customary treatment plans to find out what's best for us.

2

Midlife Crisis

o o o o o o o o o o o o o o o o o o o o o o o o o o o o o o o o o o o
The crisis of yesterday is the joke of tomorrow.

—*H. G. Wells*

We've just discussed fear and how it can affect your life. I suppose another obstacle that many of us face at 40 and beyond is the Midlife Crisis. Are you facing a Midlife Crisis? It's natural to start feeling like you're getting old when you hit 40. Of course, you don't have to feel that way and that's what this book is all about.

At age 41, Steven Johnson (not his real name) faced a problem common at midlife: His priorities were turned upside down.

"After 20 years of marriage, a business failure and a touch of depression, I just flipped and said to myself, 'To hell with it, I'm not getting any younger,'" said Mr. Johnson, a financial planner in Connecticut. He yearned to live more freely and impulsively.

The solution he chose, however, wasn't so common: restraint. Suspecting that his inner chaos was temporary, he rebuilt his career and stuck with his marriage. But, he also blended into his life some energetic pursuits that satisfy a love of adventure he had been ignoring. "I've found that one or two more weeks off by myself, and maybe a couple of weekends on a long motorcycle trip or hiking in Colorado or Arizona, go a very long way in maintaining my mental health—my sanity," he said.

Many of you may see yourself in this guy.

The term "midlife crisis" was introduced by Elliott Jacques in 1965, a psychologist and pioneer in human development theory. He found that around the age of 35 people begin to see their life in terms of "time left to live" as opposed to "time since birth," which is the previously held view.

But whether or not you specifically will experience a "crisis" during this time depends on a variety of factors. Certain aspects can make this time of life much more turbulent than it would otherwise be. These include:

- Being unhappy with your career
- Worries about the future
- Marital or relationship problems or stagnancy
- Taking care of elderly parents
- Feeling that you missed out on past experiences
- Deteriorating health

Fortunately, whether you are facing a "midlife crisis" or are looking for a new start in life for whatever reason, there are many things you can do to improve your outlook and feel great.

---

40 and Beyond Fitness Tip:

To avoid a midlife crisis, try to blend in activities that you enjoy for pure pleasure on a regular basis.

Anticipate the Problem

Spread your craziness across the decades instead of outing it all at once. Don't be undisciplined and go hog-wild, but don't suppress or repress too much either. Balance is the key.

Reassess Your Goals

Midlife is one of the best times to reassess your goals (or make them if you haven't yet). If you feel dissatisfied, first identify what it is that is causing the feeling. Then, make a specific goal to change your dissatisfaction into satisfaction.

And, be sure that when you think of goals you are not only thinking of financial ones—goals can be applied to any area of life from career to marriage to personal attitudes. Goals are an entirely personal matter, but while the process comes naturally to some it can be taxing on others. Here are a few examples of dissatisfaction and goals to change the feeling, but remember to make your goals specific to your own situation.

Dissatisfaction	Goal
Feeling Restless	Take a vacation to a new location, even if only for a day, at least once a month.
Lack of meaning	Explore at least five new spiritual, social, and/or religious outlets. The social could be a sports-related activity like joining a hiking or biking club.
Fears of children leaving home	Remember the things you enjoyed before starting a family and do them! This could include taking your wife out on a date like you used to do. Try a new activity to expand your circle of friends.

Find Interesting Projects

Find a consuming project that expresses inner desires. It could be restoring an old car, building a work area in your garage, or renovating your home.

Build Personal Relationships

As we get older, it's easy to take our existing relationships for granted and not place any importance on establishing new ones. But strong relationships with a spouse, family and friends are as important now as ever.

If you are married, make a point to refresh your routine and not take your spouse for granted and be sure to show affection if you expect to get any in return. This is easy to say and harder to do, but it is very important as your happiness and ability to be optimally productive in your life is severely limited when you are not in a happy relationship with your spouse.

---

40 and Beyond Fitness Tip:

Social ties and friends are the keys to a happy life and will become increasingly important as your children leave home.

And for everyone, whether you are married or not, be sure to actively seek and build new relationships with friends and even family members that you may have lost touch with. Social ties are one of the keys to a happy life and will become increasingly important as your children leave home and you have more time to focus on yourself.

Be Adventurous

If you're fantasizing about doing something risky, at least be mindful about it. Lise Van Susteren, a Washington, D.C. psychiatrist, advises training yourself "to evaluate risk opportunities"—to weigh dangers against the potential benefits. Dr. Van Susteren took her first bungee jump in New Zealand at age 52, and says "it was out of this world." Though she's afraid of heights, she says diving 14 stories was so thrilling it was worth the effort.

Join a Support Group

An El Paso, Texas, housing-finance specialist says he found help in several, including one run by two therapists on analyzing troublesome relationship patterns, and another offered by his church for people going through divorce.

Eat Nutritious Food

I've covered this in several areas of this book and I'll keep on discussing it at every point. It's so important, I believe in repeating it many times. You simply cannot hear too often the importance of good nutrition. Many people underestimate the power food can have on emotional health. And with a midlife crisis, much of the crisis is typically emotionally based. Eating junk food is just about the worst thing you can do during this time as sugar can cause depression and a host of other health problems. So, especially if you're having a midlife crisis at 40 or beyond, stay away from sugar!

---

40 and Beyond Fitness Tip:

Especially if you're having a midlife crisis at 40 or beyond, stay away from sugar!

Eating other junk foods or the wrong foods for your metabolic type will imbalance you not only on a physical level but also on an emotional one. This can easily leave you feeling irritable, nervous, angry, hyper, depressed or hopeless.

Similarly, the right foods will feed your body and your mind and will leave you feeling strong, energetic, in control and emotionally sound.

Consider Making a Change

If you have seriously contemplated your current situation and are not happy with it from any angle, it may be time to make a change. Now, I am not suggesting that one day, you pick up and leave your family behind or anything of that nature. However, you may want to discuss some new options with your spouse and family.

This could include changing careers, moving to a new area of the country, expanding your social connections and so on, depending on what you are looking for. The point to realize is that you do not have to stick with a sinking ship; it's O.K. to want to change some aspects of your life. You will want to be aware of those around you, however, and be sure that the ship is actually sinking before you decide to bail out. So, don't do anything rash. You must take responsibility for yourself and your family.

40 and Beyond Fitness Tip:

Recognize that it's O.K. to change some aspects of your life. This could include living arrangements, careers/jobs, and the activities that you do in your free time.

If you're having a midlife crisis, here are some resources:

- *The Third Age: Six Principles for Growth and Renewal after Forty,"* by William A. Sadler. Based on a 12-year study of successful adults in midlife.

- www.lessonsforliving.com: A clinical psychologist describes the psychological underpinnings of midlife crises and gives advice for managing them.

- www.midlifeclub.com: Resources and a good chat room focused largely on the family woes caused by midlife crisis.

- Support Groups: Contact your church or local newspaper or community center to find groups suited to your needs.

3

Slowing Down Time

o o o o o o o o o o o o o o o o o o o o o o o o o o o o o o o o
"The future depends on what we do in the present."

—*Mahatma Gandhi*
Indian Nationalist Leader

There isn't a day that goes by that I don't appreciate and value time. It's a precious gift and so many of us waste it frivolously—especially when we're in our 20s and early 30s. In our youth, we think we're going to always have an abundance of it—that it will always be at our beck and call.

---

40 and Beyond Fitness Tip:

Time is the only commodity you have that is beyond your control.

Time is the only commodity you have that is beyond your control. I am extremely grateful that I decided to take charge of my life when I did and to change my priorities. That's the only way we really can control time to any degree.

Generally, most of us don't do anything to keep "time" in check—or to minimize the effects of aging. Most of us salivate over fast cars, fast food, fast talk, and fast books. We seem to worship speed in the Western world. We don't realize that we're simply hurrying old age and opening the doors for Mortality to step in with a bear hug.

Time is closely related to Mortality because it tells us that, because we're mortal, we only have a finite amount of it. Actually, as Soul, we know we're going to live forever—just not in the physical state. So, Time does become an important

18

commodity when we're here on Earth, living our life. And, if you follow my guidelines in this book, you can *slow down time. What? You must be joking;* you're shaking your head and saying to me. *Whoever heard of slowing down time?*

But, trust me, you can do it. Since it's such an important commodity, I want you to make the best use of your time possible.

Do you know what it feels like when you start a new diet or exercise plan? How the days seem to drag on and the weeks crawl by slowly one by one? You think, *"Can I possibly make it through the week without eating sugar or having that delicious cheeseburger?"* If you think of it in terms of *slowing down time*, then you can say, "Oh, I love this. I have so much time to accomplish the things I want to do. I still have 4 more days in this week." In this way, you're slowing down time.

In Jay Griffith's brilliant book, *A Sideways Look at Time*, Jeremy P. Tarcher, 2002, she discusses a fellow in Sweden who pulled an emergency cord on a train and, when it stopped, distributed leaflets reading, "Speed is an unnecessary evil that is destroying our lives and our planet." No doubt most of the passengers were angry that he had slowed down their trip. He had, in essence, slowed down time. A growing number of people are protesting the fast pace of modern culture and our clock-dominated linear, and work-oriented view of time.

---

40 and Beyond Fitness Tip:

You can slow down time by stopping…Look at your life, rearrange your daily activities. It is possible to slow down time.

You can also slow down time by stopping and rearranging your daily routine of activity. That's right. *Stopping.* I now make a point to *stop* my daily routine and meet a friend for golf every week. We like to go to the golf course early in the morning before anyone else is up. Sometimes, it's quite chilly, so we put 2 propane heaters in the cup holders on the golf cart to keep us warm. He and I both are very busy executives and some people think we're nuts to get up so early and venture out on the golf course just as the sun is coming up. But, the truth is, we love it. We've learned how to *stop* and *slow down* time. Those early morning times are the best. It's quiet. It's slow. Each moment rolls by slowly, lazily, and methodically as if it's being perfected just for him and me. As if it's something confidential between just him, me, and the universe. And, what's even cooler is that we don't keep score. We play golf for the pure pleasure of it. No competition. Just fun. When was the last time you did something for the pure pleasure of it? And, I'm not talking about eating that chocolate cupcake…that's something that may or may not be good for you. I'm talking about something that doesn't add inches to your waistline and doesn't cost much. Something that's just for the pure pleasure of it—like watching the sun rise or set...or playing golf with your best buddy early in the morning before anyone else is awake.

It's all about prioritizing and downsizing...that's all. When you downsize your life and reorganize your priorities, you'll find that you have more time to enjoy the things you love. You'll have more time to enjoy life.

On the following page, make a list of the things you love to do just for the pure pleasure of it. Set time aside throughout the day and the week to do these things. Keep this list handy and whenever you're feeling stressed or that life is out of your control, stop and make a point to do one of those things. Observe how it slows down your life—how it slows down time—and helps you to appreciate your time even more.

Things I Love To Do

Time is Controlled By Our Thoughts

Did you know that time is mostly controlled by our thoughts? All the events you have experienced in your lifetime up to this moment have been created by the thoughts and beliefs you have held in the past. Until I hit 40, my thoughts were focused on being rich and successful, and those thoughts controlled my time.

But, that is my past. And, it can be your past too. It's over and done with. What is important in this moment is what you are choosing to think and believe and say and do right now. For these thoughts and words will create your future and control your time. Your point of personal power is in the present moment and is forming the experience of tomorrow, next week, next month, next year, and so on.

So many people focus on negative thoughts the way I did when I hit 40. I thought my life was burned out—washed up—and that I was old. I let this negative thought roll over me like a giant truck and as I did this, I was letting it control my time and my destiny. Gratefully, I had an epiphany and decided to take charge of my life. I know you can do this too. Stop for a moment and notice what thought you are thinking. Is it negative or positive? Do you want this thought to be creating your future? Do you want it to control time?

40 and Beyond Fitness Tip:

Our experiences are just outer effects of inner thoughts.

No matter what the problem is, our experiences are just outer effects of inner thoughts. Even self-hatred is only hating a thought you have about yourself. You have a thought that says, "I'm 40. I'm old. I can't do anything like I used to." This thought produces a feeling and you buy into that feeling. However, if you don't have the thought, you won't have the feeling. And thoughts can be changed, my friend. Change the thought and the feeling must go. Change the thought and take control of your time and your destiny.

40 and Beyond Fitness Tip:

Thoughts can be changed. Change the thought and take control of your time and your destiny.

You will learn as you incorporate the exercises and tips in this book that being active and healthy will give you the upper hand in the battle against the clock—against time. A consistent program of exercise and nutrition—along with re-prioritizing your life—can combat, alleviate, and even reverse some of the effects of aging. When you gain control of your body, you will more easily gain control of your life, and only then will you gain some control of time. And, guys, don't we all want more time to hang out with our families and enjoy a little football, golf or basketball?

4

A Vision & Attitude for Success

o o o o o o o o o o o o o o o o o o o o o o o o o o o o o o o o o o o o o

"Imagination is the beginning of creation. You imagine what you desire; you will what you imagine; and at last you create what you will."

—*George Bernard Shaw*

It's all in the attitude. You are in control of your destiny. If you believe it, you can achieve it. I know you've probably heard this many times, but have you ever really thought about it?

Moods

Moods, for better or worse, are an expression of your physical and psychological state. They can be triggered by emotions, brain chemistry, hormones or blood sugar, as well as by too much or too little food, exercise or sleep.

"Negative moods are like subtle indications that we need more energy," writes psychologist Robert Thayer, Ph.D. in *Calm Energy*. Thayer believes that physical activity, even in short bouts and varied intensities, is a positive tool for mood management. In fact, just 10 minutes of moderate exercise can improve overall mood, as well as increase vigor and decrease fatigue, according to a study in *Health Psychology*. And, don't we all need that in our super-stressed, super-hectic lives?

Why does this happen? There are a number of theories, including the release of feel-good brain chemicals like endorphins and serotonin; a reduction in the stress hormone cortisol; increased self-esteem resulting from better body image and weight control; and even muscle relaxation due to raised body temperature. Also, those who exercise away bad feelings are less likely to turn to smoking, overeating or alcohol, which can feed cycles of tension and depression. That doesn't mean that you can't enjoy an icy cold beer while you're watching a ballgame, or that you can't take pleasure in an after-dinner cognac. It just means that if you're depressed, then go easy on the alcohol because it will only enhance the depression.

---

40 and Beyond Fitness Tip:

Too much alcohol and smoking can feed cycles of tension and depression.

Whatever the reasons, exercise works; you can override mood swings simply by moving your body. Hear that, guys? *Get moving!* The following suggestions are related to specific temperament and behavior characteristics. Choose one that you need at a given time to positively transform how you feel.

Mood Elevators

- *Get incensed:* Oils are not just for women. Use oils, incense or aromatherapy techniques to raise your spirits or calm down. (This will also give you brownie points with your spouse or girlfriend. She will *love* seeing you be more sensitive and may want to join you in a meditative or romantic moment.)

- *Stay in the light:* Different lighting sources can affect mood. Natural light contains necessary ultraviolet rays to help regulate emotional balance, while constant exposure to fluorescent light has been known to drain energy and raise stress levels.

- *Listen:* Sounds simple, doesn't it? But, it's not always so. Sound has a profound effect on your senses and can alter your mood consciously or subliminally. Keep specific tunes at hand that will inspire, energize or relax you whenever you need it.

- *Hug a tree:* Trust me. It works. Get outside in a natural setting. You don't necessarily have to really hug the tree, but just being there will make you feel calmer and more at peace and one with nature. And, even big burly guys need this. Even a 10-minute refresher is enough to change a state of mind. Walks in a plush park are ideal.

- **_Get comfy:_** Be aware of comfort clothes, such as your favorite sweater, your sweatpants, and your boxer shorts. Whatever it takes to provide a sense of pleasure.

- **_Change the scenery:_** If your office desk is a stress-maker, reorganize it so you feel more in control. Taking a short break from a stressful situation or environment, especially between activities or tasks, will help adjust your attitude.

- **_Don't wait to exhale:_** Deep, meditative breathing can have a significant effect on your physical and mental state. "Breathing may be the master function of the body, affecting all others," writes Andrew Weil, M.D., in _Spontaneous Healing._ "How we breathe both reflects the state of the nervous system and influences the state of the nervous system."

- **_Make a List:_** Write down 10-15 things you're grateful for in your life. Smile as you write them.

Visualization

Have you ever known someone who was so passionate and emotional that nothing could stand in the way? Throughout history, people such as Thomas Edison, Henry Ford, the Wright Brothers, Bill Gates and Mother Teresa all had a passion so strong that no matter the obstacles, they made their dreams come true. What was their secret to staying so driven? How did they ignite their passion every day? They each had a very clear plan, a mental blueprint that guided them successfully to their targets.

---

40 and Beyond Fitness Tip:

You must have a blueprint, a mental plan, before you can truly achieve your goals.

You need a similar passion to build your healthy body. Having a mental blueprint is critical to your success. With a clear target, you have the most powerful advantage to making your dream body a reality. Imagine trying to build a house without a blueprint or traveling to a new place without a road map. It can't be done.

This is where visualization comes into play.

Many people may wonder what is meant by visualization. Some worry because they don't actually see a mental picture in their mind when they close their eyes and try to visualize. First of all, don't get stuck on the term "visualize." It isn't necessary to "see" an image. Some people say they can see very clear, sharp images when they close their eyes and imagine something. Others feel that they don't see anything, but they just sort of think about it or imagine they are looking at it. They also might become aware or feel an impression. That's O.K. We all use our imaginations every day, so whatever process you find yourself doing when you imagine, it's fine.

If you still don't feel sure what it means to visualize, then I'll walk you through this exercise. Guys, it's important to first visualize a trim, fit body, before you set out to attain it. Visualizing it will make it become real.

Visualization Exercise

Find a quiet spot in your house or somewhere in nature where you can be alone. I like to go to my bedroom either first thing in the morning before I start my day or right before I go to bed when the world has calmed down a bit.

Sit down, close your eyes and relax deeply. Think of some familiar room or place that makes you happy. Remember some familiar details about it, such as the color of the walls and the way the furniture is arranged. If you're thinking of the beach, visualize the blue water lapping up gently on the shore. Smell the salty sea air with white clouds floating by. Wherever you imagine, and then see yourself walking into that room or on that beach. Look at yourself. Visualize a trim, healthy, happy, lean body. *How does it feel? Strong? Good?* Let yourself really enjoy these feelings. *Feeeel* (get excited about) yourself in your new, fit, healthy, *young* body. Putting real emotion into your visualization is one way to make it become real. Do this every day for 15-20 minutes. If it helps, put on some music to help you relax. In 20-30 days you should start noticing a change in your attitude about yourself, your body and your life.

40 and Beyond Fitness Tip:

I am convinced that life is 10% what happens to me and 90% how I react to it. And so it is with you...we are in charge of our attitudes.

Charles Swindoll

You still with me, guys? I know I've thrown in a lot of interesting tidbits and motivational suggestions to help you get ready for your transformation. I've found that all these things help and at age 40, it's time to start looking in-depth at the reasons why we do or don't do things.

In the next section of the book, I'm going to focus on *"Getting Started." Enjoy!*

PART II
Establishing the Baseline

5

Check-Up Time

◆

Are You Ready?

o o o o o o o o o o o o o o o o o o o o o o o o o o o o o o o

"There's only one corner of the universe you can be certain of improving and that's your own self."

—*Aldous Huxley*

A few years ago, I was at the neighborhood gym playing basketball with a group of guys in their late 20s. This was something I did at least twice a week. After the third game, one of the guys said, "Hey, I'm gonna have to rest. I can't keep up with the rest of you young guys."

Amused, I looked at him and said, "How old are you?"

"I'm 30 years old…I'm not as young as the rest of the guys."

"Do you know how old I am?" I asked.

"Well, I'm assuming you're in your late 20s like the rest of the guys out there," he nodded toward the rest of the group.

"Nope, I'm over 40," I smiled.

"No way," he said. "You don't look a day over 30. What's your secret?"

"Lots of basketball," I laughed. "And, good nutrition—that kind of thing."

He just shook his head as if he didn't believe me and I went back out on the basketball court with even more energy than before. To be mistaken for someone in their 20s…well, you know how it is, guys. We *love* that, don't we? It's not just women who love to be mistaken for someone much younger—we guys like it too—especially after we hit the 40 mark.

31

40 and Beyond Fitness Tip:

It's not just women who love to be mistaken for someone much younger—we guys love it too!

You may even be over 40. If you consider that bad news, then I've got some good news for you. Forty is just a measurement of time—and your body doesn't have to listen. Along with leading health experts, I've designed some plans in this book to help you look and feel younger. I believe the best years of your life are ahead of you. I know mine are.

It's been said that no one can make us feel inferior without our own consent. Feeling old is the same way. Our bodies, we seem to forget, take orders from us. If we want them to be fit, firm, and feisty, they can be—and for a lot longer than perhaps our grandparents expected their bodies to be. Research now leaves no doubt that exercise can help preserve virtually every physical muscle tone and strength, bone mass, physical endurance, flexibility, resistance to disease, mental acuity, and even sexual vigor. *Hey, guys—forget about Viagra.* You won't need it as you age if you follow the plans I've outlined in this book!

The problem is that most of us simply let these capacities dwindle out of neglect. But, no longer—right?

Are you ready to get started? Are you ready to select a food plan, an exercise plan and change your life? If so, then read on.

I would like to mention that it is wise to check with your doctor before you begin any diet or fitness plan. Getting a complete physical will let you know if you have any major obstacles that you need to focus on before attempting a health and fitness plan.

6

Nutrition

✦

We Are What We Eat

∘ ∘

"Within each of us lies the power of our consent to health and to sickness, to riches and to poverty, to freedom and to slavery. It is we who control these, and not another."

*—Richard Bach, **Illusions***

Keep in mind that I am not a health practitioner or dietician. I am an ordinary guy like you who simply wants to stay as healthy as possible for as long as I live.

An article printed in the *El Paso Times* on January 17, 1996, from the Gannett News Service quoted several authorities who said the following:

Americans eat more, pass on exercise.

Despite all the badgering to eat better and exercise regularly, Americans still aren't, a new federal report shows.

People are eating more calories than they did a few years ago. And even though they're eating lower fat food, they're eating more fat simply because they're eating more. They're not eating their dark green or yellow vegetables.

On top of that, many aren't exercising vigorously.

Participants reported weighing an average of 11-12 pounds more in 1994 than they did in the late 1970s.

The Centers for Disease Control and Prevention announced in November 1998 that the high-fat, high-carbohydrate snacks that have made our teenagers obese have also triggered Type 2 diabetes. While a formal study has not yet been done, it appears that the number of these cases has tripled in the past five years. Following are some more alarming statistics:

Americans spend about $33 billion a year trying to shed pounds.

One type of cancer of the esophagus has increased more than 350 percent among white men in the past 20 years, and the researchers say the reasons may include smoking and an increase in obesity.

As for dietary cholesterol, studies demonstrate little effect of reducing intake of foods containing cholesterol in most adults and no effect in a sizable subset of otherwise healthy subjects.

Table sugar may shorten life span and increase aging. Researchers theorize that excessive sugar ultimately generates free radical chemicals that mess up proteins and accelerate the aging process, causing disease and premature death.

Some statistics from the *Journal of the American Medical Associate* indicate that one in every three adults is overweight; obesity accounts for more than $68 billion per year in excess healthcare costs and loss of income. We spend over $30 billion per year on diet foods, diet products, and diet programs; and physicians are more likely to treat the conditions exacerbated by weight gain (such as diabetes, cardiovascular disease, and hypertension) than to treat obesity itself.

It doesn't sound good, does it? Americans are simply eating more calories and we are getting fatter. We aren't getting enough vigorous exercise either. Did you ever carry a 12-pound backpack while jogging, let a lone a 50- or 100-pound backpack? When we are fat, it is too hard to exercise.

So, let's focus on what we should be eating. I am aware that there are many different diets out there on the market and I'll review them in another chapter. Right now I want to highlight the foods that I eat to stay healthy and slim. I truly believe that if you want to successfully and consistently lose weight, these are the things you must do!

---

40 and Beyond Fitness Tip:

Eat like a king for breakfast, a prince for lunch and a pauper for dinner.

---

1. **Never skip breakfast.** This is probably the single most important thing to do when trying to lose weight and stabilize your metabolism. If you're used to just grabbing a cup of coffee in the morning, you need to commit to something more right now if you want to be successful. Actually, breakfast is one of your most important meals and should be your largest, as this is what

revs up your metabolism. Forget the myth that if you eat breakfast it will stretch out your stomach and you'll eat all day. This isn't true. Only through sticking to a good, nutritious breakfast have people been able to successfully maintain their weight. Remember this: "Eat like a king for breakfast, a prince for lunch, and a pauper for dinner."

2. **Never skip a meal.** In order to lose weight and properly maintain, you have to stabilize your metabolism. This is the key to maintaining. Once you've lost weight with an efficient metabolism, you will be able to occasionally go out to eat and splurge on your old favorites without gaining. The key word here is "occasionally." You simply cannot stabilize if you tend to skip meals.

3. **Drink 8-10 glasses of water (64 oz.) daily.** This is an absolute MUST. Water suppresses the appetite. Generally speaking, the heavier you are, the more you should drink.

4. **Try not to eat after 6:30 p.m.** This is hard for many of us, but you can do O.K. eating later if you simply eat lighter. Make it as nutritious as you can. Just make it a small meal!

5. **Keep your daily fat gram intake under 30-35 grams.** This is quite simple when eating healthy. The average American eats over 65 grams of fat daily. Most of that is due to the preparation of foods (frying as opposed to grilled or baked), and those high fat condiments. Say goodbye to the oils, butters and cream sauces, and use the nonfat condiments. You'll never feel deprived and you'll cut the fat right out of your diet.

6. **Sodium.** Learn to recognize which foods are high in sodium since they tend to make you retain water, which shows on the scale. Those include teriyaki sauce, soy sauce, canned foods, fat free hot dogs, etc. Add a slice of lemon to your water as a natural diuretic.

7. **Exercise will help you look and feel better.** The benefits of exercising regularly will give you more energy, burn more calories to help you lose extra pounds, and help you maintain your weight. Exercise also tones the muscles, increases resistance to fatigue and improves self-image. Exercise will help you relax and feel less tense, so you'll sleep better. And, another added benefit is that regular exercise helps to control your appetite!

Exercising

We'll focus on exercising more in-depth in another chapter, but for right now, here are a few tidbits.

---

40 and Beyond Fitness Tip:

Exercise at least 3 times a week and build your level of fitness to exercising at least 5 times a week.

Exercising should be done in 3 stages.

1. 5-10 minute warm-up session

2. 20 minutes minimum of aerobic exercise

3. 5-10 minutes of cool-down session.

Exercise at least 3 times a week and build your level of fitness gradually.

Some Healthy Substitutes

Following is a good food plan—the kind I enjoy in my daily life. I've listed it for you so you can see the choices I make. However, everyone's body is different and unique, and what may work for me, may not necessarily work for you. I urge you to check with your doctor and then experiment with different diets to see which one is best for you. Following this chapter is a whole section devoted to comparing the different popular diets on the market. You may find one of those diets more suitable for you than what I've listed here.

Meat & Substitutes

You have 4 choices each day totaling 400 calories. (100 calories per serving). The point is to have no more than 1,500 to 2,000 calories daily and only 30-35 fat grams daily. Remember, add 64 oz. of water, too. Plus, always try to buy organic meats, fish, fruits and vegetables if possible.

- 2 oz. Cooked poultry—skinless

- 1 oz. Lean beef (round, sirloin, flank, tenderloin)

- 1/4 cup tuna (water packed)

- 1 oz. Lean veal (chops or roast)

- 1/4 cup dry soy bean product

- 2 tbs. Grated parmesan cheese

- 3 egg whites

- 1 oz. Lean pork

- 2 oz. Fish or shellfish

Fruit

You may select 4 choices each day at 60 calories per serving, totaling 240 calories daily.

- 1 fresh medium fruit (apple, pear, peach, nectarine)

- 1 banana (6 inches long). Only one allowed per day

- 1 cup berries or melon

- 1/2 cup canned fruit (in juice without sugar)

- 1/4 cup dried fruit

Vegetables

Make sure your vegetables total 100 calories for the day.

- Steamed or raw (as desired

Milk

You have 3 choices each day at 90 calories per serving, totaling 270 calories daily.

- 1 cup nonfat milk or nonfat yogurt (frozen is O.K.)

- 3/4 cup 1% fat milk

- 1/2 cup 2% fat milk

- 1/3 cup powdered milk before adding water

- 1 Jello fat-free pudding (any kind)

- 1/2 cup 1% cottage cheese

Starches/Bread/Grain

You have 4 choices each day at 80 calories per servicing, totaling 320 calories daily.

- 1/2 cup pasta or barley

- 1/3 cup rice or cooked dried beans or peas

- 1/2 cup starchy vegetable (corn, limas, potato, peas, squash)

- 1 slice whole grain bread (2 slices of 40 calorie bread is O.K.)

- 1/2 bagel (any kind)

- 1/2 English muffin

- 1 tortilla (6 inch corn or flour)

- 3 cups popcorn (air popped)

- 4-6 crackers (rye crisp or saltine type)

- 1/2 cup whole grain cereal.

Following these nutritional guidelines you will receive approximately:

20% protein

60-60% carbohydrates

Less than 25% fat

Things to Remember

1. Watch portions. Even fat free calories count!

2. If you fall off one meal, get back on track the next meal—not the next day. And, don't beat yourself up about it. Move on.

3. Prepare foods using the 4 Bs:

    Broil

    Bake

    Boil

    Barbecue

4. No fried foods! Cook with Pam. Canola and olive oils are the best choices of oil, but they still have 14 grams of fat per tablespoon, so use sparingly.

5. Read labels carefully. And, don't be fooled by labels. They are based on 2000 calories.

Fresh Fruit Exchanges

Fruits

Select either fresh, frozen or canned in water or own juice. When selecting fresh fruit, try to always select organic whenever possible. Keep in mind that fruit juices contain too little fiber and too much sugar!

Apples	1 small
Applesauce	1/2 cup
Apricots	4 raw
Banana	1/2 (6 inches long)
Blackberries	3/4 cup
Cantaloupe	1/3 melon
Cherries	12 raw
Figs	2
Fruit cocktail	1/2 cup canned
Grapefruit	1/2 medium
Grapes	15 medium

Honeydew	1/8 melon
Kiwi	1 large
Mango	1/2 mango
Nectarine	1
Oranges	1 medium
Papayas	1 cup
Peach	1 fresh or 3/4 canned
Pear	1 small or 1/2 canned
Persimmon	2
Pineapple	3/4 cup or 1/3 cup canned
Plum	2
Pomegranate	1/2
Raspberries	1 cup
Strawberries	1 1/4 cup
Tangerine	2
Watermelon	1 1/4 cup

Dried Fruit

Dates	3 1/2
Prunes	3 medium
Raisins	2 Tsp.

Vegetables

Select either fresh, frozen or low sodium canned products.

Artichoke

Asparagus

Bean sprouts

Beets

Broccoli

Brussel sprouts

Cabbage

Carrots

Cauliflower

Celery

Cucumber

Eggplant

Green beans

Green pepper

Greens (collard, mustard, turnips)

Okra

Onions

Snow Peas

Spinach

Summer squash

Tomato

Turnips

Vegetable juice (1/2 cup low sodium)

Zucchini

7

Comparing the Top Diets & Trends

The world over, we're trying to make peace with our meals as we struggle at the most extreme ends of the feast-or-famine spectrum. Science is working overtime to solve our culinary problems: Fat mice are made skinny at the tweak of a gene. We have more data than ever before about life threatening French fries and cure-all blueberries. And rice, corn, wheat, and other crops are now engineered to resist drought and produce abundantly.

Super-sized drive-thru dinners and the off-kilter global distribution of food illustrate the daily struggle to be good to ourselves and good to each other. We overlook the fact that eating lunch at 40 miles per hour while driving back to work doesn't qualify as nurturing the body. We overlook the hunger for love and care shared by the starving child in Africa and the obese child in America. We're so often living mindlessly that we miss these connections between body and soul. I know I was. Before I had my epiphany on my 40th birthday, I just ate on the run. I was too busy making money to stop and really nurture my body with the right foods and nutrients.

Cleansing & Detoxification Diet

Even though I am not a health care professional, I know that we're all concerned with health and wellness. And, we all know that we're not getting sufficient nutrition in our foods today. Following are some dietary and health recommendations as general guidelines that have been associated with cleansing and detoxification programs. The following food plan is especially good for any of you who have had some serious illnesses or diseases, or for those with compromised immune systems. Specific health situations may require that individuals receive guidance from their physician. Please bear in mind that these recommendations are not intended to diagnose, treat, cure or prevent disease.

1.   Drink plenty of fluids (1 liter = 1quart +) for every 50 lbs. of body weight). Pure water is of extreme importance to maintaining proper balance and remaining healthy. Most people complain about having to drink water, but you simply cannot become healthier without it. Do not expect long-term success without proper hydration.

2.   Your cleansing diet should contain no more than 20-25% protein per meal. You may choose from low stress proteins such as tofu, soaked nuts and seeds, chicken, turkey, fish, and eggs. Organic or free range is ideal. Shellfish are often discouraged by practitioners since many are found to contain harmful bacteria and mercury.

3.   75-80% of your cleansing diet ought to come from the foods listed on the following page. These are alkalizing and cleansing foods which will help support the rejuvenation process. Vegetables should become your new best friend. They protect against microform overgrowth and mycotoxins, as well as help neutralize acid in the blood and tissues.

4.   Eat raw (raw, if you have strong digestion) or lightly steamed vegetables in order to maintain their active enzymes. Heating over 118 degrees destroys enzymes which is why you want to consume a lot of your food raw—or at least cooked as little as possible. During the cleansing cycle, we like to make use of a diet rich in enzymes, chlorophyll and phyto-nutrients.

5.   Foods to AVOID:

   a.   No nuts (unless pre-soaked), corn, cheese, milk, wheat. Many people have developed food sensitivities or intolerances to certain kinds of foods. Corn contains 25 different mycotoxin-producing fungi, including carcinogens. Peanuts contain 26 carcinogens. Dairy and egg products contain hormones, steroids, antibiotics, microforms, mycotoxins and pesticide residues. Plus, they are acid-forming.

b. No artificial sweeteners. Aspartame (Nutrasweet), saccharine (Sweet and Low), neotame, sucralose (Splenda), acesulfame (Sunette, Sweet & Safe, SweetOne), and cyclamates. They are all acidifying. Stevia, an all natural sweetener, is the only thing I would recommend.

c. No microwaved foods. Microwaving denatures food.

d. No caffeine, sodas, sugar and fried foods. They produce acid in the body.

6. Make sure you chew your food well. This gives the digestive process a chance to extract all the value from food. Chew 20-30 times with each bite of food.

7. Keep a positive outlook on life and share your experience with your friends and family.

8. Make sure to participate and be involved in something greater than yourself.

Low Stress Foods:

Almonds	Figs, dried	Pineapple
Apples	Grapefruit	Prunes
Apricots	Grapes	Quinoa (grain)
Artichoke	Green beans	Radishes
Asparagus	Honeydew melon	Raisins
Avocado	Kale	Raspberries
Bananas	Leafy greens	Rhubarb
Beans, Dried	Leeks	Rutabagas
Beets	Lettuce	Sauerkraut
Beet Greens	Lemons	Spinach, raw
Blueberries	Lima beans, dried	Strawberries
Broccoli	Lima beans, green	Sweet Potatoes
Blackberries	Limes	Tangerines
Brussels sprouts	Milk, goat's	Tofu
Cabbage	Millet	Tomatoes

Carrots	Muskmelon	Watercress
Cantaloupe	Okra	Watermelon
Cauliflower	Onions	Zucchini
Celery	Oranges	
Chard leaves	Parsley	
Cherries, sour	Parsnips	
Collard greens	Peaches	
Cucumbers	Pears	
Dandelion greens	Peas, green	
Edamame (non-GMO)	Peppers, green	

Other Food Items and Condiments that Alkalize:

Bio or Celtic Sea Salt (table salt is No good)	Miso
Ghee (purified butter)	Rice Syrup (has no gluten)
Olive oil	Seaweed—Kombu, Hijiki, etc.
Bragg's Liquid Aminos	Xylitol
Bragg's vinegar	
Pure maple syrup	
Molasses	

The Zone Diet

The idea behind this diet is that your digestive system operates ideally when eating just two food groups: lean protein and natural carbohydrates, like fruits and fiber-rich vegetables.

- According to the Zone Diet, the ideal ratio of carbohydrates, proteins, and fats is 40-30-30, respectively.

- The five fingers of your hand should remind you to eat at least five times a day; three meals and two snacks.

The Atkin's Diet

The foundation of the Atkin's Diet is a four-phase eating plan, combined with vitamin and mineral supplementation and regular exercise.

- **Phase 1**: Referred to as "Induction." This first step involves restricting daily carbohydrate consumption to 20 grams, obtaining carbohydrate primarily from salad and other non-starchy vegetables.

- **Phase 2**: "Ongoing Weight Loss" (OWL) In Phase 2, Atkin's dieters add carbohydrate, in the form of nutrient-dense and fiber-rich foods, by increasing to 25 grams daily the first week, 30 grams daily the next week and so on until weight loss stops. Then subtract 5 grams of carbohydrate from your daily intake so that you continue sustained, moderate weight loss.

- **Phase 3**: "Pre-Maintenance." Make the transition from weight loss to weight maintenance by increasing the daily carbohydrate intake in 10-gram increments each week.

- **Phase 4**: "Lifetime Maintenance." Select from a wide variety of foods while controlling carbohydrate intake to ensure weight maintenance.

The South Beach Diet

Like the Atkin's Diet, the South Beach Diet plan is divided into phases.

- **Phase 1**, which lasts 14 days, is the strictest. You eat normal-sized helpings of lean protein, such as chicken, turkey, fish, and shellfish. Vegetables are also allowed, so are nuts, cheese, and eggs. The goal is to eat three balanced meals a day, and to eat enough so that you don't feel hungry all the time. A typical South Beach Diet breakfast is two eggs and lean bacon.

- **Phase 2**, which lasts until you reach your weight-loss goal, allows you to reintroduce some foods that are banned in phase one, such as whole-grain breads and low-fat dairy foods.

- **Phase 3** focuses on weight maintenance. It should be used to maintain your healthy weight. Dr. Agatston, the cardiologist who created the diet, describes this phase as a "way of life." Should your weight begin to climb, you repeat the diet plan.

How Low Carb Diets Work

How does a low carb diet work? Certified personal fitness trainer James Cannone gives the lowdown on these popular diets:

He says that cutting carbs will cause you to lose weight, but not much actual body fat, if any at all. So, why do most people lose weight so quickly? It's because the human body holds 2.4g of water for every 1 gram of carbohydrate consumed. Cut the carbs and all you do is hold less water! This artificial weight loss is the main reason so many people are going low-carb.

So, not only does following a low-carb diet cause you to lose water, it also depletes muscle glycogen which leaves you feeling sluggish when trying to be active or work out. Remember, carbs are stored as glycogen in the muscles and glycogen is what's used to fuel your muscles.

Another problem with severely limiting carbs is that the brain uses carbs for energy and without enough carbs, you won't be 100% mentally fit. While Cannone agrees that people are different and that some people do better on lower amounts of carbs, most people will feel like crap after a week or two with no or low carbs.

Low-Carb Diets Giving Fruits a Bad Reputation

"The intake of fruits and vegetables has been too low for a long time," Dr. David Katz, a professor at the Yale University School of Medicine and the nutritional columnist for *O: The Oprah Magazine,* says. "It was too low before Atkins. Those diets are causing a problem even if they're not reducing the intake of vegetables very much, and that is distracting people from the absolutely critical importance of increasing both fruit and vegetable intake. They actually have some people convinced that eating fruit is bad for them, and that's wrong."

A Pioneer of Low Carb

Dr. Richard Mackarness, author of *Eating Dangerously: The Hazards of Allergies,* Harcourt Publishing, 1976, and who promoted an Inuit-style, meat-only diet, and the doctor who ran Britain's first obesity and food allergy clinic says:

- A person's metabolism falls into one of two distinctive types, the constant-weight, always-slim type, and the fatten-easily type.

- Weight gained by people in the latter group is due to an inability to break down carbohydrates fully because of a metabolic defect, and not as the public at large believe, because of weak-willed gluttony.

- Man's problems with obesity began 8,000 years ago, with the advent of cereal planting. For 4 million years before that, man was a hunter who survived by killing and eating meat, which has led to complete biological adaptation to a meat diet, but not to a cereal diet, because it is too recent.

Anything that the Stone Age man would have eaten is going to be good for people with the fatten-easily type of metabolism, whereas anything of cereal origin (especially if refined or processed) will cause weight to be gained. Refined white flour is described as the worst culprit, and Mackarness quotes Doctors who consider it so pernicious that it should be sold with a Government Health Warning, like cigarettes.

- **Carbohydrates**—should be kept as low as possible, and in any event must not exceed 60grams per day for the majority of people. In some cases, 50grams per day or even less may be necessary.

- **Protein and Fat**—both of these should be high, with a ratio of 3:1 respectively by weight.

- **A Fast**—of up to a week is recommended as a prelude to all diet attempts, unless there is a medical contra-indication.

Mackarness lists 6 pages of foods with their protein and carbohydrate values, and symbols alongside each entry indicating whether they can be taken freely, in moderation, with great caution or not at all. He is very keen to keep food varied and interesting, and provides specimen meals for a whole week.

Typical Menu:

Breakfast

- Half a grapefruit, or fresh orange juice.

- Fried bacon and eggs, using preferably the cheaper streaky cuts of bacon.

- Or ham, either with omelette or scrambled eggs, made using plenty of butter

- Kippers, Bloaters or Haddock, (the latter stewed in milk). Or kidneys, or liver.

- Tea with top of the milk, or coffee with cream and no sugar

Lunch

- Beef stew with vegetables in it, but no flour thickening. Alternatively, vegetable broth, un-thickened.

- Any of the following: corned beef, mince, ham, tongue, tuna fish, sardines, pig's head brawn, fried sprats, boiled skate, pilchards in oil, whelks, winkles, jellied eels, or any fish without batter.

- Wedge of cheese or cheese souffle, salad or green leaf vegetables, or peas or French style green beans, with butter.

- Fresh fruit, or unsweetened rhubarb, with cream.

- Coffee, with cream but no sugar.

Tea

- Cheese, nuts, apple, yogurt, cup of tea with top of milk

Dinner

- Bowl of consomme or clear soup

- Half a pound of meat with its fat: lamb, beef, bacon, ham, pork, veal, "flank," liver or breast of mutton

- Tomatoes, lettuce, cauliflower, cabbage, spinach, peas, head of braised celery, watercress

- Cheeses and fruit (apple, orange, plums, pineapples, etc., but not bananas) and cream.

- Nuts.

- Tea or coffee, black, or with top of the milk, or with cream

Nightcap

- Wedge of cheese or hard-boiled eggs. Cup of hot oxo, bovril or marmite.

Unique Features:

Exercise:

This was considered at length. Mackarness finds evidence both in favor of and against exercise, and leaves choice to the reader.

Fat:

Consumption of dietary fat is actively encouraged. The author states that, "In the absence of carbohydrates, fat is not fattening".

Sugar:

To be removed from diet. Certain artificial sweeteners can be used if absolutely necessary.

Protein:

Emphasis on fresh, unprocessed meat, fish and poultry, supported by other permissible foods.

Other Notes:

Several aspects of this book and diet have more recently been covered by the book, *Neanderthin.* The author's references to "top of the milk" were made prior to homogenized milk, in the days when each pint of milk had a layer of cream at the top of it.

The Fat Flush Plan

The book titled, *The Fat Flush Plan,* by Anne Louise Gittleman was published in 2002, but the first fat flush eating plan made its debut in her book, *Beyond Pritkin,* released in 1988.

Anne Louise Gittleman is one of the most respected, dynamic, and accomplished "celebrity" nutritionists America has ever produced. As a writer, consultant, talk show host and spokesperson, Ann Louise has imprinted her distinctive message on everything she does.

Emphasis is not given solely to controlling insulin production, but to "Five Hidden Weight Gain Factors" being:

- Liver toxicity

- Waterlogged tissues
- Fear of eating fat
- Excess insulin
- Stress fat

The ratios in Gittleman's Fat Flush Plan resemble the Zone's—40/30/30. The plan has three set guidelines:

- **Phase 1**: The two week Fat Flush
- **Phase 2:** Ongoing fat Flush
- **Phase 3:** The lifestyle eating plan

Phase 1 is the toughest stage of the program and has been labeled "Boot Camp." It is first and foremost a cleansing program to facilitate weight loss by giving the liver support and nourishment.

Phase 2 is designed for ongoing weight loss with a bit more variety in food choices adding back a friendly carb each week to check for adverse reaction to it.

Phase 3 is really the Fat Flush maintenance program providing a lifelong eating program aimed at increasing your vitality and wellbeing for life. At this time, 2 dairy products can be reintroduced and a variety of starchy veggies and non-gluten grains. Once again, new foods are added back one at a time to gauge your body's reaction. Once on this stage of the program you will likely find your daily percentages work out at the ratio 40:30:30.

The Fat Flush Plan is made up of whole natural foods eaten without salt. You have to eliminate trans-fats, caffeine, diet sodas, alcohol, aspartame, sugar, yeast related vinegar (except apple cider vinegar), all grains and cereals, starchy vegetables, in the first phases dairy products (except whey) are also cut.

Flaxseed oil (2 tablespoons) and an essential fatty acid supplement are to be taken daily. One cup of unsweetened cranberry juice is to be watered down to make up 64 oz. and taken throughout the day.

First thing upon waking and last thing at night you are to take a teaspoon of psyllium husks in a glass of the cran-water, dubbed the "Long life cocktail." Gittleman recommends lemon juice in the morning in a cup of hot water, up to 8 oz. of lean protein a day and 2 eggs a day. You may choose an unlimited amount of vegetables from the non-starchy, low glycemic index section. You can also have up to 2 fruits a day from the low glycemic index, like 1/2 grapefruit or one cup of berries.

Typical Menu

A Day on Phase 1: The 2-Week Fat Flush Plan

Try this sample menu.

On rising:

Long Life Cocktail

Before breakfast:

8 ounces hot water with lemon juice

Breakfast:

Veggie scramble: 2 scrambled eggs with spinach, green peppers, scallions and parsley, and one 8-ounce glass of cran-water

Midmorning snack:

1/2 large grapefruit

20 minutes before lunch:

One 8-ounce glass of cran-water

Lunch:

4 ounces of salmon with lemon and garlic, warm asparagus, mixed-green salad with broccoli florets and cucumber, 1 tablespoon flaxseed oil, and one 8-ounce glass of cran-water

Mid-afternoon:

Two 8-ounce glasses of cran-water

4 p.m. snack:

1 apple

20 minutes before dinner:

One 8-ounce glass cran-water

Dinner:

4 ounces of grilled lamb chop with a pinch of cinnamon and a dash of dried mustard, sautéed kale in broth, baked summer squash with a touch of cloves, and 1 tablespoon flaxseed oil

Mid-evening:

Long Life Cocktail

How to Use This Menu:

You can use this example as a basic menu guide. Just substitute foods from the same food groups for daily variety. Besides the daily diet, take GLA supplements, and a balanced multivitamin/mineral. You can change the fluid intake to suit your schedule if that is more convenient, of course.

Unique Features:

No herbs or spices except for those fat flushing herbs and spices outlined in *The Fat Flush Plan*

No margarine

No alcohol

No sugar

No oils or fats except those in the flaxseed oil

No grains, bread, cereal or starchy vegetables such as beans, potatoes, corn, parsnips, carrots, peas, pumpkin, or acorn or butternut squash

No dairy products

How to Pick Your Diet Plan

Here are some general guidelines for who will do best on each type of diet.

You'll do best on a low-fat diet if you....

• Don't eat a lot of meat.

- Enjoy fruits, vegetables and whole grain foods.

- Need volume to feel full.

- Eat meals regularly—about every 4 to 5 hours.

- Don't travel or eat out frequently. (Fresh fruits and veggies and whole grains can be hard to find, and restaurants tend to use lots of fat.)

- Have high cholesterol.

- Are willing to have your cholesterol levels checked. (If they go up, which they do for some people, this is probably not the right diet for you.)

You'll do best on a calorie-counting diet if you....

- Need a lot of variety.

- Don't mind measuring portion size.

- Find yourself standing in front of the refrigerator trying to identify the food you are craving.

- Can eat only a little of something you like.

- You have given up on diets because you were bored with the foods they offered.

You'll do best on a low-carbohydrate diet if you....

- Enjoy eating meat, cheese, and eggs.

- Find it hard to feel full without eating these foods.

- Don't care much about variety.

- Are able to limit fruits and vegetables.

- Can say goodbye to breads, pastas, and sweets.

- Travel or eat out a lot. (You can always find meat or fish and a salad, the prototypical meal of this diet.)

- Are willing to have your cholesterol levels checked. (If your triglycerides go up, which they do for some people, this is probably not the right diet for you.)

I wanted to give you some basic diets and food plans as a way to help you get started on your *"Fitness after 40 Plan."* Again, we are all different and you may want to experiment with these diets and see which one is best for you. What works best for me might not necessarily work best for you and vice versa.

8

Vitamin Supplementation

✦

Do You Need It?

○ ○

The right questions precede the right answers.

As any doctor will tell you, lack of energy is one of patients' most common complaints. The food and beverage industry knows this, as consumers spend billions a year on products loaded with caffeine and sugary carbs. While these stimulants may get you out the door in the morning and on your way, you may as well by hopping on a Harley with a broken fuel tank.

After caffeine and sugars ratchet up your blood sugar, your body releases a flood of the hormone, insulin, which makes sugar levels sink. Within an hour or two, fatigue and hunger return, and you reach for another cup of Joe and something sweet. So goes the speed-crash-and-burn cycle.

There's a better path, one that leads to steadier, healthier highs. Several nutrients—coenzyme Q10, alpha-lipoic acid, carnitine, ribose, and certain vitamins—work with your body's natural processes to provide physical and mental energy at the cellular level. They naturally increase the activity of your mitochondria, tiny cell structures that break down glucose and fat and convert them into the chemical form of energy, known as ATP. Supplementing with these critical nutrients can lead to higher, more sustained energy levels. Here's how they work:

- **Coenzyme Q10:** Made in limited amounts by the body, coenzyme Q10 helps shuttle around energy-carrying electrons in the mitochondria. In 1985 researchers at the University of Texas reported that patients suffering from cardiomyopathy, a life-threatening weakening of the heart muscle, improved significantly after taking coenzyme Q10 supplements. Since then, dozens of clinical studies have confirmed the nutrient's full-body energizing effects. By strengthening the heart muscle, coenzyme Q10 helps it pump blood and nourish cells throughout the body. This can also help your skin look younger and more vibrant.

- *Vitamin E:* According to a study presented at the American Association for Cancer Research's annual meeting, taking vitamin E once a day may lower your risk for prostate cancer by up to 53%. Meanwhile, despite earlier claims to the contrary, a new report from the Medical University of South Carolina found that taking grape-seed extract may not reduce your risk of developing cancer. Researchers say the disease-fighting antioxidants found in whole foods like grape juice and wine appear to lose their effectiveness in pill form.

- *Honey:* New research from the University of California, Davis, reported that eating honey may help protect you from toxins in the air, lowering your risk of heart disease and cancer. In trials, researchers found that men and women who ate honey regularly had higher levels of disease-fighting antioxidants in their blood than people who rarely ate the sweet stuff.

- *Alpha-Lipoic Acid:* Alpha-Lipoic Acid is a potent antioxidant that also boosts energy levels. It works in two principal ways. It improves the body's response to insulin, helping to burn blood sugar; this results in more stable blood sugar and insulin levels, which help prevent energy dips and hunger jags. It also revs up the energy-producing activities within mitochondria, leading to higher ATP levels in the body and the brain.

- *Conjugated Linoleic Acid:* The most compelling CLA research to date—in both people and animals—focuses on its ability to reduce body fat, build lean muscle mass, boost resting metabolic rate, and maybe even make dieting a little more pleasant. Studies show that it won't miraculously help you lose weight—you still need to diet and exercise for that—but once you've shed some pounds, CLA can help keep you from gaining them back as fat. According to the researcher, Michael W. Pariza, Ph.D., he discovered that CLA thwarts an enzyme that allows fat to pour into fat cells, preventing them—and you—from growing larger. In a new study, researchers put 60 overweight men on a restricted diet to make them lose weight, then told them to resume their old eating habits with one small change: Half the group was asked to take CLA, the other half, dummy capsules. After 13 weeks, both groups regained weight, but for the men who took CLA, more of it came back as lean muscle, not flab. (Muscle weighs more than fat.) More muscle boosts the rate at which you burn calories at rest, making pounds come off more easily.

- **Carnitine:** A nutrient found in animal protein, carnitine helps transport fats through the mitochondria and into the chemical reactions that convert them to energy. It is especially beneficial for those with chronic fatigue syndrome (CFS). In one double-blind study on CFS patients, carnitine was shown to improve energy levels and reduce pain significantly. But, it can boost energy in otherwise healthy people, too.

  In a recent animal study, a combination of carnitine and alpha-lipoic acid increased the energy output of mitochondria, improved memory, and doubled the level of physical activity. According to the study, the improvements were comparable to giving a 70-year-old person the physical and mental vigor of a 40-year-old. Human trials are currently under way. But, this can be very encouraging for all of you 40+ guys!

- **Omega-3 Fatty Acids:** This important nutrient promises less cardiovascular disease; lower risk of lethal heart attack; depression relief; better brainpower in old age; less risk for cancer, and improvements in rheumatoid arthritis and asthma. Traditional sources of Omega-3s have dried up. Beef was once a rich source because cattle grazed on grass, which is full of Omega-3s. But, today's grain-fed beef doesn't have any. Since your body can't make essential fatty acids, you need to consume them. Salmon, tuna, sardines, mackerel, and other fatty, cold-water fish are full of them. If you're not a fish fan, then opt for supplements. To find the best quality supplements, see test results from the independent supplement evaluation lab, ConsumerLab.com.

- **Vitamin C:** Vitamin C is best known for enhancing immune function and reducing cold and flu symptoms. But the first physical signs of vitamin C deficiency are fatigue and irritability, according to a landmark study by the National Institutes of Health. Vitamin C is needed for the body's synthesis of carnitine, and low levels of either nutrient interfere with the burning of fats for energy. Some research suggests that vitamin C supplements might improve endurance among athletes.

- **B-Complex Vitamins:** B-vitamin deficiency is a frequent culprit in low energy, particularly among vegetarians who may not get enough B12 in their diets. Several of the B-complex vitamins play crucial roles in the breakdown of blood sugar and fats to generate energy. In particular, vitamins B2 (riboflavin), B3 (niacinamide), and pantothenic acid play key roles in what cell biologists call the energy-generating Krebs cycle. The B-complex vitamins are also considered to be antistress vitamins, protecting against moodiness and irritability. To reduce the chance of causing an imbalance among the B-complex vitamins, it's always better to take them as a group rather than individually.

- ***Ribose:*** Ribose forms the carbohydrate backbone of DNA and RNA, and it is also a key building block of ATP. As a dietary supplement, large amounts can improve strength and stamina, particularly among people involved in regular physical activities. A study at the University of Florida, Gainesville, found that bodybuilders taking ribose increase their bench-press strength and the number of repetitions they could complete, compared with those taking placebos.

---

40 and Beyond Fitness Tip:

Supplements should not replace healthy, whole foods.

Supplements, of course, should never replace healthy foods. But, with the commercialization of food and produce grown on soil sterilized and poisoned with pesticides and herbicides, our foods have lost their nutrient density and therapeutic value. Add to that our drugged, caffeinated society and modern lifestyle that includes over-medication, chlorinated water, environmental pollution, and a stressfully fast pace, it's no wonder we've lost our vitality, energy, and good health. The result is that people are now more susceptible to disease and illness than ever before. One of the best ways to compensate for these unhealthy stressors is to supplement our diets with essential nutrients and nutrient dense foods. In other words, it's time to take self-responsibility for our health and wellness.

Supplements probably won't provide maximum benefits if you continue eating fast foods and a lot of sweets and refined grains.

To sustain your energy levels, aim to stabilize your blood-sugar levels and minimize the extreme up and down swings that leave you tired. You can do this by eating more lean protein and fiber-rich vegetables and cutting back on carbohydrate-rich convenience foods, including breakfast bars, pasta, muffins, bagels, and soft drinks.

And, don't forget to sweat. Going for a 30-minute walk or bicycle ride several times a week helps lower and stabilize blood-sugar levels. And the more you exercise, the more muscle you will build and this will help your body burn glucose and fat efficiently.

Of course, remember—whatever diet you choose may not be the one I'd choose and vice-versa. You have to listen to your own body's needs to determine which diet is best.

Finally, it's important to remember the bromide about not burning the candle at both ends. When you are consistently tired, your body is telling you something. Pay attention. Listen to it, and keep in mind that, more often than not, the best medicine is a good night's sleep.

9

Water, Water, Everywhere...

◆

The Body's Need for Hydration

Goals and actions must meet.

—*Sir Winston Churchill*

Drink more spring or filtered water to improve every facet of your health. You've heard it repeatedly: Make sure you drink at least eight 8-ounce glasses of water per day. The key words are "at least" because, unless you are a child or the size of a child, you need more water than that. The rule of thumb is, for every 50 pounds of body weight you carry, drink one quart of bottled spring or filtered water per day. The average person weighs 150 lbs., so they should drink three quarts per day. A 200 lb. person should drink a full gallon per day. Athletes should drink even more than that. Follow these guidelines and you've successfully adopted one of the most crucial health habits.

Our bodies are mostly water, and so this ongoing intake of water is essential to our every function. Drink the appropriate amounts, and everything is much more likely to function at optimal levels. Don't drink enough water, and over the short term you will experience routine fatigue, dry skin, headaches and constipation; over the longer term, every body function will degrade more quickly. It really is as simple as that.

Things get a bit more complicated in what type of water to drink. Bottled spring water and filtered water are both good options. Do not drink tap water or distilled water. The spring (not "drinking") water should be bottled in clear polyethylene or glass containers, not the one-gallon plastic (PVC) containers that transfer far too many chemicals into the water. Filtered water can be obtained through low-cost filters, such as those provided by Brita or PUR brands. Another recommendation by some of the leading healthcare practitioners is the GE Smart Water, which was top rated in *Consumer Reports*, December 2002.

Tap water should be avoided because it contains chlorine and may contain fluoride, toxic substances that, with ongoing consumption, can have dire consequences for the body. Distilled water should also be avoided because it has the wrong ionization, pH, polarization and oxidation potentials, and can drain your body of necessary minerals. It has been tied to hair loss, which is often associated with certain mineral deficiencies.

Finally, drink water at room temperature if possible, as ice-cold water can harm the delicate lining of your stomach. Your body needs an absolute minimum of six to eight 8-ounce glasses of water a day. Alcohol, coffee, tea and caffeine-containing beverages don't count as water.

---

40 and Beyond Fitness Tip:

Water is the cheapest form of medicine for a dehydrated body.

The best times to drink water are one glass one half hour before taking food—breakfast, lunch, and dinner—and a similar amount two and one half hours after each meal. This is the very minimum amount of water your body needs. Naturally, if you work out, you need to drink more water continually throughout your workout to keep your body hydrated. For the sake of not short-changing your body, two more glasses of water should be taken around the heaviest meal or before going to bed.

Thirst should be satisfied at all times. With increase in water intake, the thirst mechanism becomes more efficient. Your body might demand that you drink more than the minimum 8 glasses a day.

Adjusting water intake to mealtimes prevents the blood from becoming concentrated as a result of food intake. When the blood becomes concentrated, it draws water from the cells around it.

The extensively researched and fascinating book, *Your Body's Many Cries for Water*, by F. Batmanghelidj, M.D., should be required reading by all, and definitely belongs on every person's bookshelf who is interested in improving his/her health.

Now that I've gotten you prepared and ready, it's time for some action. Read on, my friends. The time has begun!

PART III

Get Ready...Set...Action!

◆

Exercises & Thoughts to Keep You Young

10

Exercising

o o o o o o o o o o o o o o o o o o o o o o o o o o o o o o o o o o o o

Every day in every way I'm getting better and better.

—*Emile Coue*

"Not enough time" is the number one reason people give for not getting more exercise. Things get in the way. Like getting the kids off to school. And working. And your son's soccer practice. And taking the lawnmower to the shop to be repaired. And spending time with your spouse.

But it is possible to save a few minutes of your day and week for a workout. To help you figure out where those minutes are in your busy schedule, I've designed some time-management tips and strategies to help you work in exercising.

The Centers for Disease Control and Prevention reviewed over six decades of research and found that stretching does little to prevent injury during exercise when done outside of a warm-up. In some cases, the increased flexibility that stretching promotes may actually impede performance.

Many physicians and exercise physiologists agree that rigorous bouncing, an early incarnation of the stretching and flexibility trend that took root in the 1970s, is not the way to go. Most experts say the bouncing, or ballistic stretching, is more likely to cause injury than other forms of it.

Rather than stretching before physical activity one can do the sporting activity at 50 percent of the target intensity for a warm-up.

Exercising is a critical component to maintaining good health, especially as you age.

When planning an exercise program it is helpful to have a guide.

---

40 and Beyond Fitness Tip:

Exercise is critical to maintaining good health, especially as you age.

Here are some key points to remember when exercising:

- Make exercise a priority. This one is key. All other strategies pale in comparison. The most successful exercises simply make exercise a top priority, says University of Georgia exercise scientist Patrick J. O'Connor, Ph.D. They put it on their daily "to do" list and stick to it.

- Schedule workouts in advance. It's best not to make training decisions on a day-to-day basis. You can always modify your weekly schedule if something comes up, but it's important to set the initial framework. And be sure to check with your family before engraving anything in stone.

- Remember why you exercise. Remind yourself that it's for your health and happiness—and no, that's not selfish. Because exercise gives you more energy for work and non-work activities alike, everyone benefits, not just you.

- Create a survival workout. For days when you just don't have time, Stan James, a Eugene, Oregon-based orthopedist, recommends devising a 15-minute "survival workout" that allows you to maintain momentum. The particular activity doesn't matter. Just keep it simple and "at the ready" for when its' needed—because it will be.

- Learn to squeeze exercise into even the tightest spots. For example, if you have to take the car into the shop to be repaired and have to wait for an hour, go walking or running for that time.

- Make your commute active. If your office building has a shower or you don't mind sponging off in the men's room, consider running, walking, cycling, or skating to work. Of course, this requires planning ahead for a change of clothes. And you may need a ride home via a friend or public transportation if two self-powered trips are too many in one day. Perhaps the homebound commute is more feasible. Pack your exercise clothes, ride to the office with your spouse or friend, and when 5 o'clock comes, run, walk, cycle, or skate home. You can stuff your office attire into a duffle bag or store it in your office and retrieve it another day.

- Park and walk. If commuting to work really isn't practical, consider driving and parking a mile or so away, then walking the rest of the way.

Remember that you'll have to walk the same distance after work as well, so be aware of time constraints.

- Work out first thing in the morning. You might find it difficult at first, but once you get used to it, you'll find you have so much energy throughout the day that you'll be hooked.

- Work out during lunch. Put fitness before food at lunchtime. Go for a walk or get in a 30-minute strength-training workout. You're likely to find that it gives you a lot more pep than a big meal. You'll need to eat at some point, of course, so just pack a healthful lunch and eat it at your desk. And, why not suggest to clients or colleagues that you take a business lunch on the road? Talk while you walk and either grab a bite at your firm's cafeteria or pick up some healthful takeout on your walking route.

- Work out before dinner. Exercising before eating can be a great way to take the edge off your appetite.

- Exercise at home. Get an exercise video, buy a cardio machine (treadmill, stationary bike, rower), or set up a weight room in your basement. That way, you can work out in the convenience of your own home. You can exercise while you watch your favorite TV shows or listening to music. Allow yourself a couple of hours to wind down afterward before going to bed—an exercise buzz doesn't generally make for the most restful sleep.

- Include the kids. With a running stroller, you can run or walk and give the little one a fun ride at the same time. Better still, play with your kids—kick ball, throw a Frisbee, play tag. Or go cycling or skating together. You'll improve your fitness and bond with your kids.

- Find a friend. One way to make certain that you fit exercise into your busy schedule is to find a training partner or two who'll depend on you to show up for a walk or a fitness class.

40 and Beyond Fitness Tip:

Listen to your body. If an exercise is hurting you and you feel pain, don't do it.

Following are some more tips and guidelines for exercising.

- Listen to your body. If exercise worsens symptoms, modify your program or stop, if need be. As your energy and health improve, you will be able to tolerate larger amounts of the aerobic exercise, which will lead to weight loss.

- It helps to hire a personal trainer who can guide you through the specifics of a good exercise program. If you do use a personal trainer, please be aware that many don't understand the nutritional principles discussed in this book.

- Be consistent. You will need at least 30 minutes of exercise a day before you will start to experience any weight loss benefits. Large studies have shown that 60 minutes a day would be better. Ideally, the exercise should be continuous, but it could be split up into two 30-minute sections.

- Start with walking if you are overweight. Most heavy people start with walking and that is an excellent choice, as it is low-risk and inexpensive. The major problem with walking, however, is that many people become fit relatively rapidly, but don't increase the intensity of the workouts as they become more fit. Once you become comfortable with a routine, it is important to increase the intensity in order to continue benefiting.

- Increase your intensity regularly. Ideally, you should exercise at an intensity that makes it somewhat difficult to talk to the person next to you. This prevents you from having to measure your pulse or use a heart-rate monitor. If you can comfortably talk to the person next to you, you aren't working hard enough to produce the benefits you need to lose weight. However, if you are using so much oxygen with your exercise that there is not enough left over to allow you to carry on a conversation then you are exercising too hard and need to cut back a bit.

- Try race walking. When outdoors, it is sometimes difficult to walk fast enough to get to this level of exertion. You can try race walking, and the web site, www.racewalk.com has an excellent section on teaching you how to do this. However, if you use a treadmill you can easily increase the incline to improve the intensity of the walking.

- Try running. If you feel ambitious you can advance to running. It is one of the most efficient and inexpensive ways to stay healthy; you don't require any equipment except a good pair of shoes. If you do decide to run, please recognize that most shoes will not last more than six months. If you use them longer than six months you will increase your risk of injury.

One of the downsides of running is that you will need cooperation with the weather. You can always use a treadmill, but that would mean the increased expense of a health club or equipment for your home. If you are elevating your program to that level, I believe that the elliptical machine is far superior to the treadmill in providing an optimal aerobic exercise experience.

- Try an elliptical machine. Elliptical machines are generally less expensive and far quieter than treadmills and provide a complete lower body workout by rotating the use of the different muscle groups on your legs. However, you will have to be sure to use the elliptical that can incline throughout various levels. Some models have a fixed base and handles that allow you to exercise your arms, but I believe it is more helpful to exercise the different leg muscles as they are much larger than your arm muscles.

You could adjust the resistance setting and frequency of steps per minute so one is just short of not having enough breath to carry on a conversation. This is the aerobic threshold that will produce cardiovascular benefits. The ellipticals are also great for reducing the boredom and monotony of exercise. What you might want to do is change the incline setting every minute or two by one notch. This will activate different leg muscles. Also, reverse the direction of the leg movement—with ellipticals, it is equally easy to walk backward or forward. You can also avoid holding on to the sidebars, which will exercise your kinesthetic sense of balance.

- Be cautious. If you are going to use exercise for weight loss you will want to consider a weight bearing exercise. It has been my experience that non-weight bearing exercises like swimming and bicycling are not as efficient or effective for weight loss. You will typically need to exercise four times as long in these activities to receive the same benefit of running or using the elliptical. Since most of us are seriously time-pressured, these exercises become less valuable for most of us.

- Swim, but only in fresh water if possible. Swimming poses the additional challenge of exposing you to the large amounts of chlorine that are in most swimming pools. However you still have the option of swimming in the lake, river or ocean depending on the temperature of the water.

- Try bicycling, but be aware of safety measures. If you decide to try bicycling you will need to be aware of the risk of injury. You can be seriously hurt on a bike so please be sure and always wear your helmet.

Sure, all these tips are great, you might be saying, but I just don't have the energy that I used to have. Well, read on and I'll explain how to get that energy high!

11

Finding Your Energy High

o o o o o o o o o o o o o o o o o o o o o o o o o o o o o o o o o o o
No opportunity is ever lost. Someone else seizes the ones you missed. ~
—*Unknown*

So, you're 40 and beyond and you just don't have the energy you used to. You're tired. Life has worn you down. Don't know if you can make it to the sofa and lift the remote. *Guys—wake up! You're still young. What are you thinking?*

Barring any serious medical condition, it's possible for just about everyone to boost overall energy levels. I'm not talking about the rush you get from downing a double espresso or the quick surge that helps you sprint a few blocks to catch the bus or train. The key to finding more energy is to build the type that really lasts. Stamina, or physical endurance, is what makes the critical difference in how much you can do from one day to the next, like logging extra miles no your stationary bike, or cleaning out the basement after a full day's work. Very simply, it's how long you're able to continue a physical activity before exhaustion forces you to stop.

Some experts believe more stamina also translates into greater mental fortitude and brainpower. "It makes sense that if you have a high level of physical endurance, you have more energy left over to devote to both physical and mental tasks," says cardiologist James Rippe, director of the Rippe Lifestyle Institute in Shrewsbury, Massachusetts, and author of *Fit Over Forty*.

Exercise and proper nutrition are the cornerstones of any stamina-building scheme—no surprise there. But something you may not know is that shaking up your daily routine can be important, too. "Introducing variety into your life can bring you more energy," says Judith Orloff, an assistant clinical professor of psychiatry at UCLA and author of *Positive Energy*.

Pump Weights and Your Lungs

Exercise is, hands down, the best prescription for beating fatigue and boosting energy. An active person loses only 1 percent or less of his physical endurance yearly, compared to 3 percent for sedentary folks. So, remaining physically active can significantly slow age-related decline. In fact, a previously sedentary person can see a 15 to 20 percent increase in endurance by exercising consistently for about 3 months.

Exercise is effective because it creates long-term changes to muscles and cardiovascular health. With regular aerobic exercise, your heart strengthens and pumps more oxygen to the muscles, prompting your body to make extra capillaries, the thin blood vessels that bring oxygen to all your cells. And the more oxygen your cells get, the hotter your internal engines can run, thereby increasing the energy production. Exercise also makes muscles produce more mitochondria, tiny engines that convert blood sugar into usable fuel. The more mitochondria we have, the more energy each cell has at its disposal.

Some form of strength training is essential: The more muscle you build, the bigger the engine you have to power your efforts. It also shifts your metabolism into higher gear, which itself is invigorating.

Action Plan

Whether it's swimming, cycling, walking, or some other heart-pumping activity, the best exercise is the one you enjoy enough to do regularly. It takes most people about six to eight weeks of working out for at least 30 minutes three to five times a week to achieve any real change in energy. Aim for getting your heart rate to your target zone (subtract your age from 220 and multiply the result times 0.6 and 0.8 to get a range). And, of course, before starting a weight-lifting program, consult a professional trainer at a fitness club, who can help you avoid injury.

Energy Waste

Don't waste energy on stuff you don't care about. Setting priorities so you fit in the things most important to you can send your energy levels soaring. "If you're not doing what you want," says Tony Schwartz, president of Resync, Inc., a corporate coaching firm and author of *The Power of Full Engagement*, "you constantly have to spend a certain a mount of energy—not even consciously—in the process of rationalizing or denying your behavior."

Even if our jobs aren't as meaningful as we'd like them to be, we all can find something in our lives that resonates with our most cherished values—whether it's volunteering for a cause, connecting with friends, or simply living as healthfully as possible—and devote some of our energy to it. The payoff, Schwartz assures, is a sense of purpose and engagement that replenishes energy instead of draining it.

Find out what's important to you by asking questions like, "Who am I at my best?" "Whom do I admire deeply?" And, "Why do I admire them?" Then, look at your schedule for a typical month to see how your priorities are reflected in what you do and start making changes. If what you value is serving others, for instance, then care out some time to volunteer.

Take Several Breaks Daily

Though our culture imposes our schedules on us, we humans are physiologically programmed to swing between spending and regenerating energy. This cycle operates in 90- to 120-minute periods during waking hours. If we ignore that pattern, we easily grow restless, irritable and tired, which depletes our energy levels. We need to shift from living our lives like marathoners and expending energy continuously, to living like sprinters who fully engage for short periods and then recover. This will boost your energy levels.

---

40 and Beyond Fitness Tip:

Instead of just surviving, we need to thrive.

So, instead of going full throttle for 8 hours, take time-outs every hour and a half or so. Take a short walk, listen to music, or meditate for a few minutes. Anything that allows you to disengage and change channels will help restore your energy.

Energy Vampires

We all know them. People who zap your energies. People can either give you energy or sap it. So, choose who you spend time with wisely. Pay attention to whether you feel better after seeing someone, or do you feel much better only after that person's gone. Draining personalities are "energy vampires." These also include the "Blamer," one who frequently faults others for her or his problems. Then, there's the Drama Queen, who goes through life at a high pitch, and the Sob Sister or Brother who keeps you on the phone for two hours complaining. Recognize these people and don't let them get to you. Remember, you can be compassionate without carrying other people's pain.

All of these tidbits will help you find your "energy high."

12

Going to the Gym

If you want to keep well as you get older,
adopt the "use it or lose it" philosophy.

O.K., I've got you guys revved up, right? You're ready to head out to the gym or somewhere to begin your fitness plan. Following are a few precautions though that you need to know about. According to a survey of 3,000 American Council on Exercise (ACE)—certified fitness professionals, there are some common mistakes you should avoid making in the gym.

- Not enough stretching. ACE recommends stretching 30 minutes, three times a week, but says that even a few minutes after a workout can make a difference. Just make sure your muscles are adequately warmed up before starting your stretching routine.

- Lifting too much weight. Only lifting what your muscles can handle is a safer and more effective way to increase muscle strength.

- Not warming up prior to exercise. Start your workouts slowly and gradually build intensity so your muscles have time to adjust to the activity.

- Not cooling down after a workout. Just as you gradually increase intensity when you begin a workout, it's equally important to gradually decrease intensity toward the end.

- Exercising too intensely. Sustained, moderate workouts are more effective than short, intense workouts, say ACE professionals.

- Not drinking enough water. Drink water throughout your workout, even if you're not thirsty. Thirst indicates that you're already partly dehydrated.

- Leaning heavily on a stair-stepper. Doing this is hard on the wrists and the back. Instead, lower the intensity enough so you can maintain good posture while only lightly resting your hands on the rails for balance.

- Not exercising intensely enough. You know you're working hard enough if you've gotten your heart rate up and developed a light sweat.

- Jerking while lifting weights. This can cause strain or injury to your muscles, especially in the back muscles.

- Consuming energy bars and sports drinks during moderate workouts. These products are high in calories and are only necessary if you're working out for more than two hours a day.

No Pain, No Gain for the Gut

O.K., 40 and older guys, we need to talk about that gut of yours. We know you're not proud of it. You may crack jokes about how you're aiming for a gold medal at the Olympics. But other than the impressive column of water you spew with each cannonball, you know that belly of yours isn't doing you any good. You don't like looking at it in the mirror, women are turned off by it, and children ask if you have a baby in there.

40 and Beyond Fitness Tip:

Big bellies don't look good on anyone.

You have more trouble sleeping than you used to, your lower back hurts, and exercise makes your knees ache. Sorry to tell you, but the problem is actually worse than that. Much worse. You see, the fat around your belly is different from fat elsewhere in your body. It's metabolically active tissue that actually functions like a separate organ, releasing substances into the rest of your body that, in excess, can increase your risk of disease. Yeah, you got it: Your own belly could be poisoning you.

Gut-Check Time

The notion that abdominal obesity is the most dangerous kind isn't new. Back in the 1940s, the French physician Jean Vague observed that some obese patients had normal blood chemistry, while some moderately overweight patients showed serious abnormalities that predisposed them to heart disease or diabetes. Almost always, the latter patients carried their fat around their middles. And, almost always, they were men.

Multiple studies since then have shown that abdominal fat—the cause of the classic apple-shaped body—is more than nature's way of telling you that you'll never become a soap-opera star, news anchor, rock legend, or Men's Health cover model. It's a sign that your body chemistry is seriously out of whack. There are a number of substances your bloated belly secretes to your heart, liver, and other vital organs. Among them are the following:

- **Free fatty acids.** Released directly to the liver, they impair your ability to break down insulin, which over time can lead to diabetes.

- **Cortisone.** High levels of this hormone are associated with diabetes and heart disease.

- **PAI-1.** This blood-clotting agent increases your risk of heart attacks and strokes.

- **CRP.** This protein inflames blood vessels, making them more susceptible to artery-clogging plaque.

The upshot of all these chemicals floating around is big trouble for big-bellied guys. In a study at the University of Alabama at Birmingham, researchers took 137 men of all ages and sizes and used seven different measurements to determine their risks of cardiovascular disease. The single best sign of multiple heart-disease risks? No, it wasn't the guys' family histories or their cholesterol profiles. It was the amount of abdominal fat they carried.

---

40 and Beyond Fitness Tip:

Heart disease and diabetes are only two of the ways belly fat can ruin your health. There are many more!

By the way, heart disease and diabetes are only two of the ways belly fat can ruin your health. If you count them all up, you'll find at least 39 different diseases associated with abdominal obesity (40, if you include looking lousy with your shirt off).

Can diet alone help you lose belly fat? Probably. In a 2000 study in the Annals of Internal Medicine, a group who only dieted dropped just as much weight (16+ pounds) and just as much belly fat (about 2 pounds) as the group who simply exercised. That said, the combination of diet and exercise is still the best ticket to permanent gut reduction. The diet-only group in the above study lost less total fat and more muscle than the exercise-only group. What's more, another, very scary study in Obesity Research looked at people who had each lost 14 pounds on a 28-day crash diet. Five years later, they had regained all the weight, with a twist: All the new weight was fat, whereas they'd originally lost a combination of fat and muscle. And their health had deteriorated in multiple ways, including increased insulin resistance and higher LDL cholesterol.

So what's the best kind of exercise for losing your gut? The short answer is any kind that you'll actually do. But intriguing new research suggests that for many guys, particularly big guys with big bellies, weight lifting may be the best way to lose weight.

In a study published in *Preventive Medicine*, researchers separated a group of people by overall build—thinner or thicker—then put them on a 12-week weight-training program. More slender guys didn't get much benefit from weight lifting, but the guys who were big to begin with gained about 3+ pounds of muscle. The implication: Bigger guys benefit most from weight training.

40 and Beyond Fitness Tip:

Bigger guys benefit most from weight training.

If you prefer to exercise on a bike or running trail, well, you'll get no argument from me.

But, if you're a weight's guy, then head for the weight room. The goal is to increase energy expenditure while building muscle. Successful gut reduction through weight training combines these two elements. You need to burn calories to lose weight now, and you need to build muscle to increase metabolism and prevent future weight gain.

If you want to shrink your gut, get enough protein in your diet. In this case, about 25 percent of calories. Why? For starters, protein makes you feel full and helps you build muscle (which increases metabolism, thereby making it easier to lose weight). Just as important, high-protein diets have been shown to be the best way of attacking belly fat. Consider a 1999 study published in the International

Journal of Obesity. Danish researchers put 65 people on either a 12 percent protein diet or a 25 percent protein diet. The low-protein dieters lost an average of 11 pounds, which isn't bad. But the high-protein subjects lost an average of 20 pounds—including twice as much abdominal fat as the low-protein group.

Get enough fat. About 30 percent of your calories. First, fat helps you feel fuller longer between meals, slowing your appetite. Second, it provides essential fatty acids needed for optimal health. Above all, fat makes you feel that you're eating real food, not starving in the land of plenty. Deprivation? Hey, man, you don't need no stinkin' deprivation.

---

40 and Beyond Fitness Tip:

You need essential fatty acids for optimal health.

If you get enough protein and fat, your total calorie intake should take care of itself. Because you feel full, you won't binge on a can of Pringles and blow your calorie count for the day. The remaining 45 percent of calories should come from carbohydrates—enough to give your palate a full range of tastes and your body a combination of fast- and slow-burning fuel.

Great Popping Pecs

So, you want to make your chest bigger? You need to "surprise" your muscles. The key to adding mass to any large muscle group, such as the chest, is varying the type of stress you put on it," says Michael Y. Seril, N.S.C.A.-C.P.T., owner of Michael Seril Fitness, a personal-training company in Orange County, California. "Try combining these two movements into one exercise," he says. It's sort of a "press-fly." The bonus: You'll save time, because you'll be doing more work with less rest between exercises.

- Lie face up on a bench, holding dumbbells with an underhand grip at the sides of your chest.

- Press the weights straight up and rotate them until your palms are facing each other.

- Keeping your elbows slightly bent, lower the dumbbells outward in an arc, chest height.

- Use your chest to pull them back up, following the same route in reverse. Lower the weights back to the starting position. That's one repetition. Perform three or four sets of eight to 12 repetitions.

13

Exercises to Live By

o o o o o o o o o o o o o o o o o o o o o o o o o o o o o o o o o
Behind every great idea are people lined up saying "it won't work."

Flatten Your Belly in 6 Simple Moves

Complete two sets of 12 repetitions of each exercise two or three times a week for the first 3 weeks; three sets of 10 repetitions of each exercise two or three times a week for weeks 4 through 6; and four sets of eight repetitions of each exercise twice a week for weeks 7 through 9.

Twist

Lie on a ball and hold a weight plate with your arms straight above your chest. Now turn your shoulders to one side, then the other.

Deadlift

Stand with two dumbbells hanging in front of your thighs. Bend forward at the hips until the weights are at about mid-shin level and your torso is as close to parallel to the floor as possible. Pause, then press your heels against the floor as you lift your torso back to the starting position.

One-Arm Rotational Row

Grab a low cable pulley with your right hand, with your right knee and left foot on the floor. Pull the handle to your right hip. Finish your reps, then switch to your left side.

Dumbbell Front Squat to Press

Stand holding a pair of dumbbells at shoulder height, with your elbows down and your palms facing each other. Lower yourself into a squat until the fronts of your thighs are parallel (or nearly so) to the floor. Pause, then drive the weights up and over your head while you straighten your legs. Return to the starting position.

Crunches

Lie on your back on an exercise ball, holding a weight plate behind your head. Raise your head and shoulders and crunch your rib cage toward your pelvis. Pause and slowly return to the starting position. You can also do this while holding the weight overhead, with your arms straight.

Lose Your Layers of Flab

Perform the workout below 3 days a week, incorporating the variations on days 2 and 3. The variations ensure that you work your muscles in a slightly different way each time, which forces you to work harder while strengthening your body at every angle—key in preventing sports injuries. Do the exercises as a circuit, moving from one to the next without rest. Complete a total of four circuits, resting 60 seconds after each.

SQUAT

Day 1: Hold one 20-pound dumbbell with both hands at arm's length in front of your body, your upper arms pressed against your chest. Keep your torso upright and lower your hips until your thighs are at least parallel to the floor. Pause 1 second, then rise to a standing position as you rotate your upper body to the left and lift the weight toward the ceiling, keeping your arms straight as if swinging a golf club. Lower the weight as you return to the starting position. Repeat, this time rotating to your right. Do 15 repetitions on each side.

Day 2: Perform the same move with two light dumbbells, holding one in each hand. As you stand up and rotate to the left, keep your right arm down while lifting your left arm toward the ceiling. As you rotate to the right, keep your left arm down and lift your right arm toward the ceiling.

Day 3: Same as day 2, but as you lift one arm, punch across your body with the other.

JUMP

Day 1: Stand with your feet shoulder-width apart and knees slightly bent. Dip your knees and jump forward as far as you can. Land on both feet with soft knees. Pause, then jump again. Complete a set of 10.

Day 2: Hop forward about 2 feet. As soon as your toes touch the floor, jump again. Complete a set of 10.

Day 3: Same as day 1, but after each broad jump, squat slightly and quickly explode straight up, reaching both arms overhead. Land with soft knees, then jump forward again. Complete a set of 10 broad jumps with a vertical jump after each.

SWISS BALL PUSHUP

Day 1: Get into pushup position with your shins on a Swiss ball and your hands on the floor. Do 20 standard pushups.

Day 2: Same as day 1, but lift one leg off the ball and do 10 pushups. Change legs and do another 10.

Day 3: Same as day 1, but move your hands out so they're 6 inches farther apart than normal.

Raising the ABS Bar

STOP CRUNCHING

With an 18-pounder, you can build abs and work your whole body. Do this program 3 days a week, resting a day in between. Complete eight to 12 repetitions of each exercise as a circuit, moving between exercises without rest to complete four circuits.

SINGLE-ARM ROW

Day 1: Stand with your knees slightly bent and hold a BodyBar or weights in your right hand with a neutral grip (palm facing your body). Lean forward at the hips until your torso is at a 45-degree angle. Pull the bar to just below your rib cage, then lower it to the starting position.

Day 2: Hold the bar in front of your right leg, palm toward you (an overhand grip). Bring your elbow up and out as you raise the bar.

Day 3: Perform the Day 1 move on one leg. Stand on your right leg and lift your left leg in front as you lean over and row.

SINGLE-ARM PRESS AND BEND

Day 1: Stand holding a Barbell above your right shoulder in a neutral grip with your right hand. Press the bar up until your arm is straight. Bend to your left side. Pause and return to the starting position.

Day 2: Dip your knees slightly. Quickly push the bar up while standing up. Pause, then lower the weight.

Day 3: Same as Day 2, but jump in an explosive movement. Land on both feet, but with your opposite foot (left if the bar is in your right hand) forward and leg slightly bent, and back leg straight.

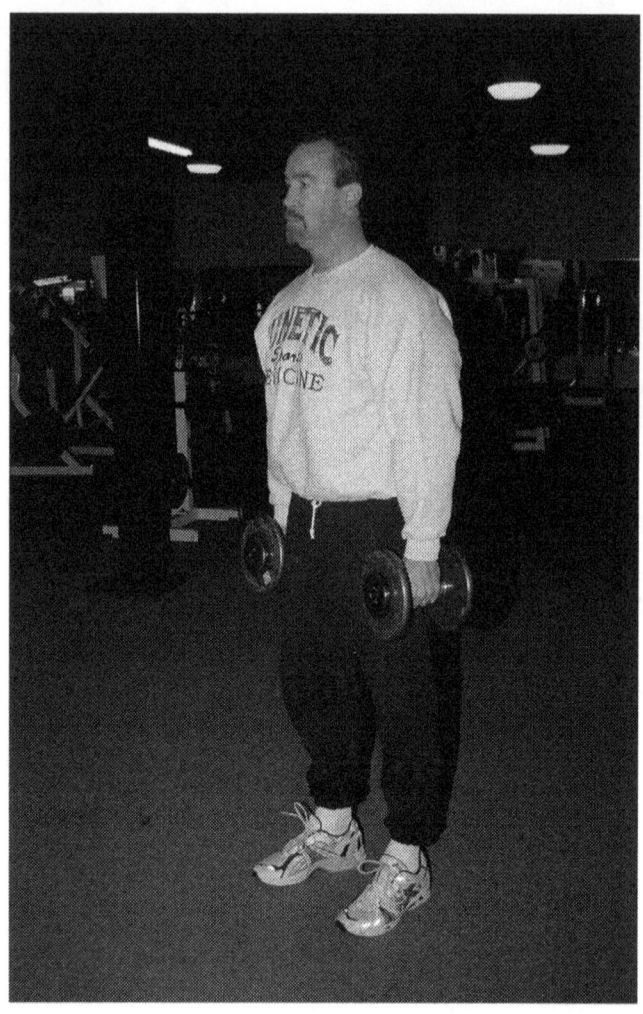

Photos courtesy of Bartolo-Vasky Photography Inc.
Thanks to Seth at Safari Gym in Phillips Ranch, CA.
Photos of Dr. Dave Martin, my chiropractor and best friend.

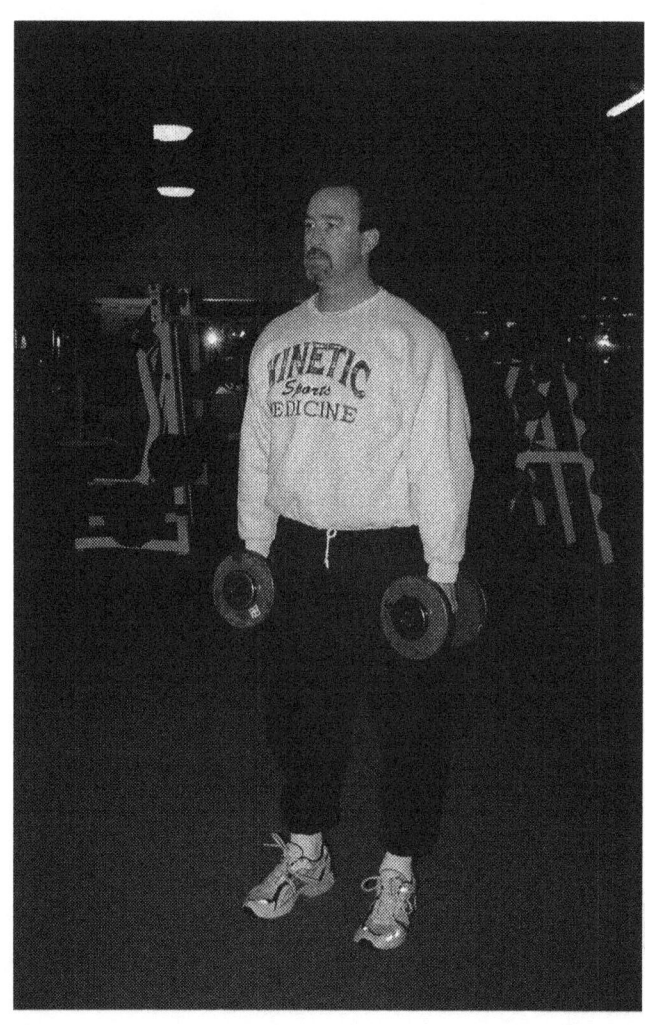

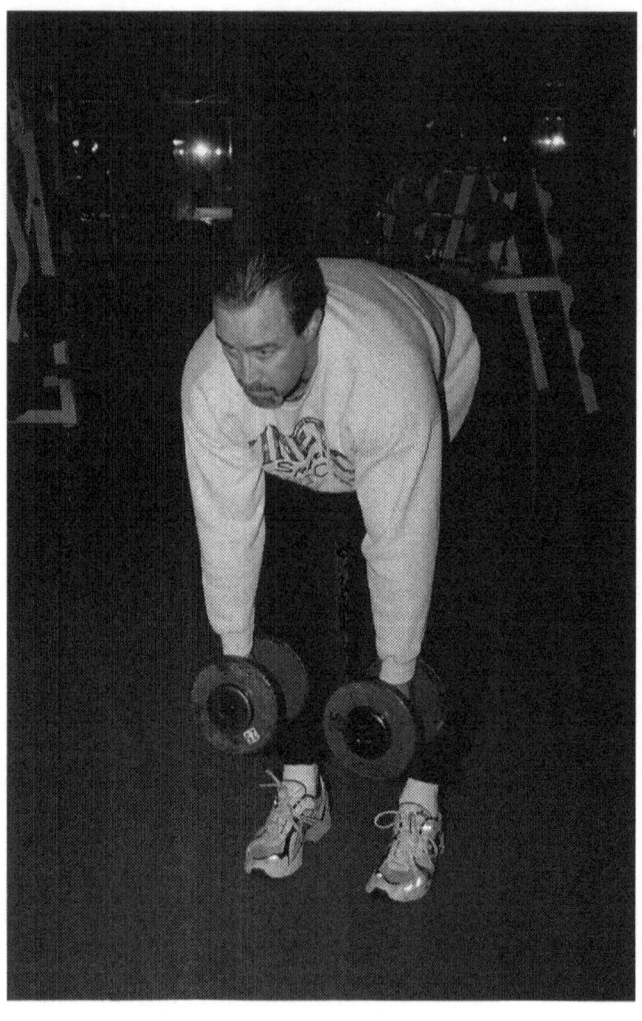

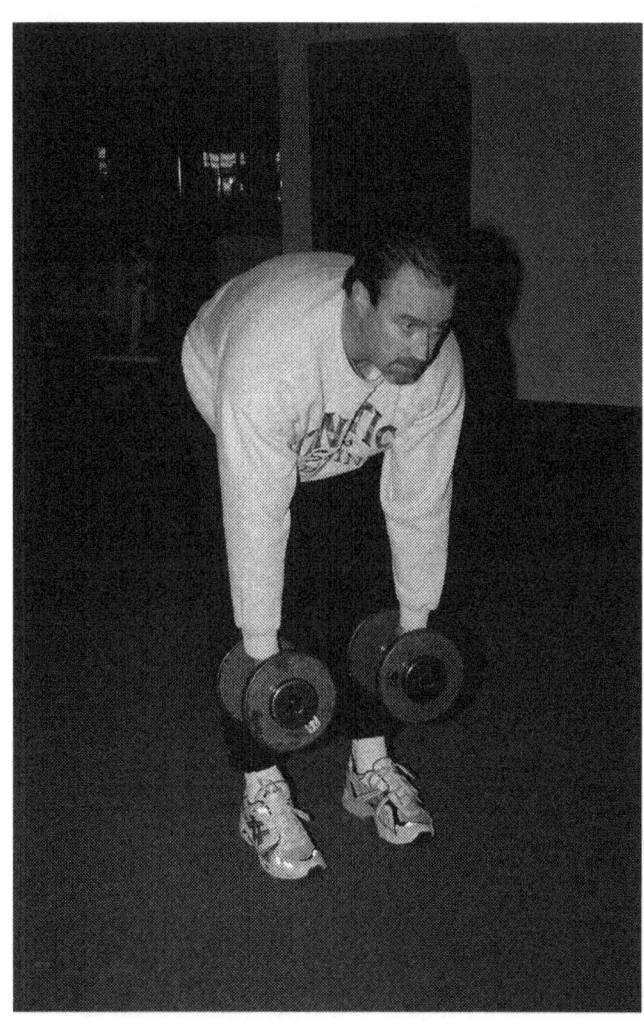

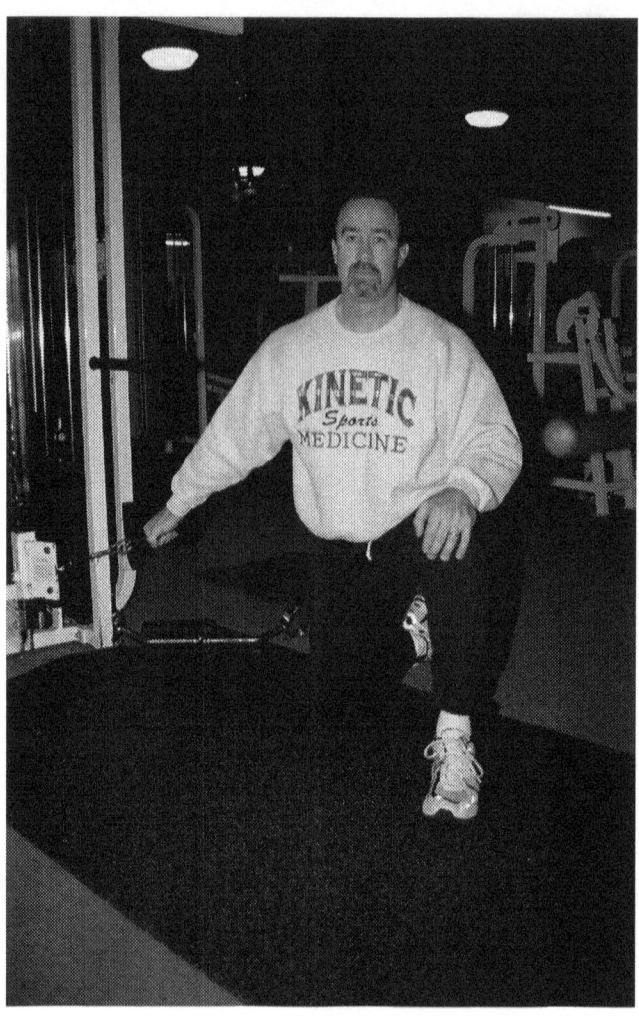

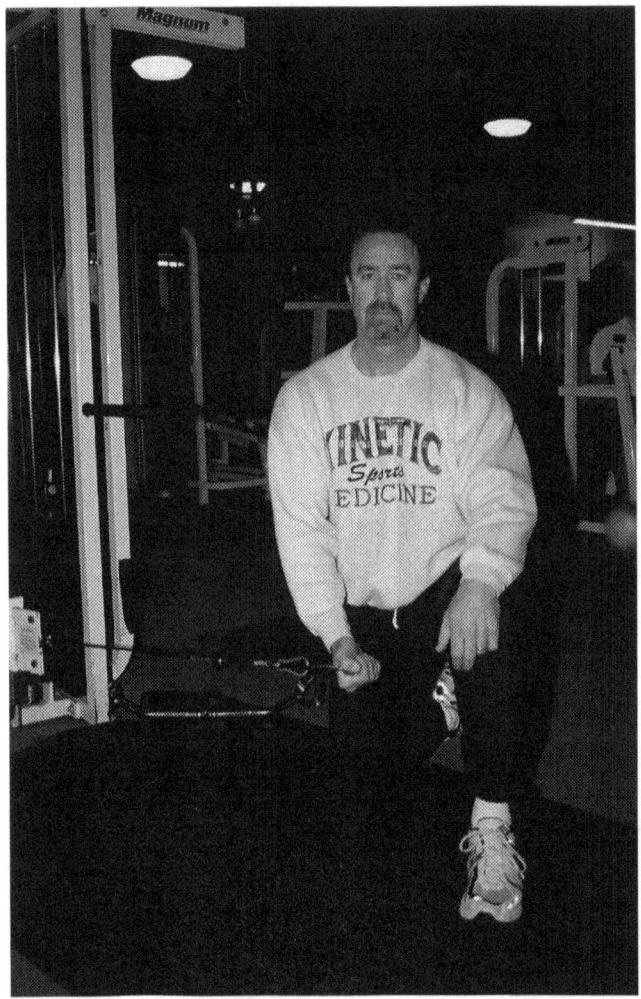

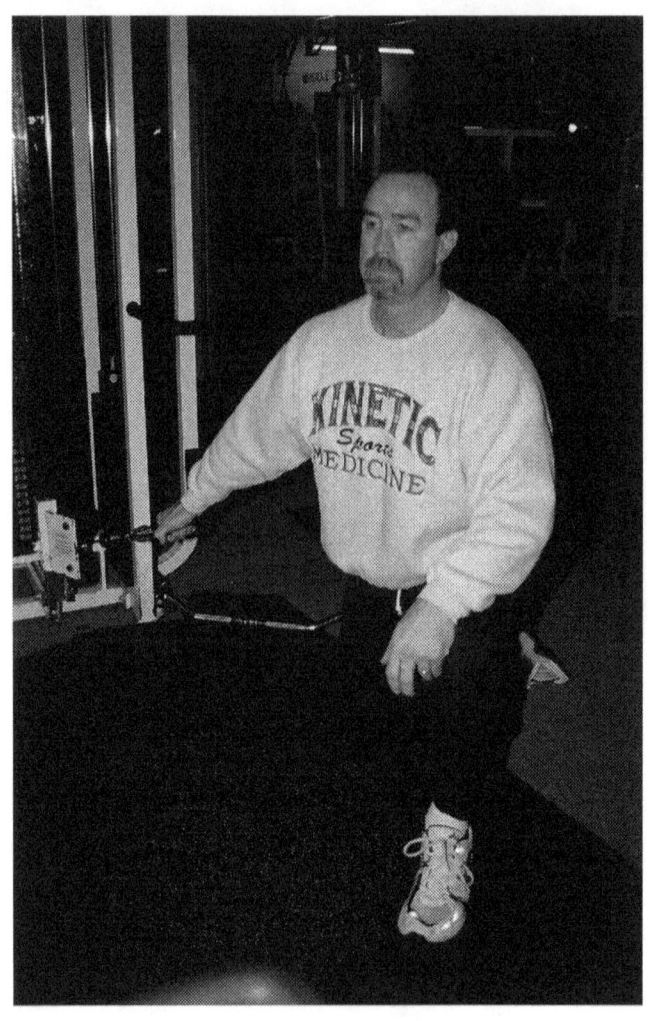

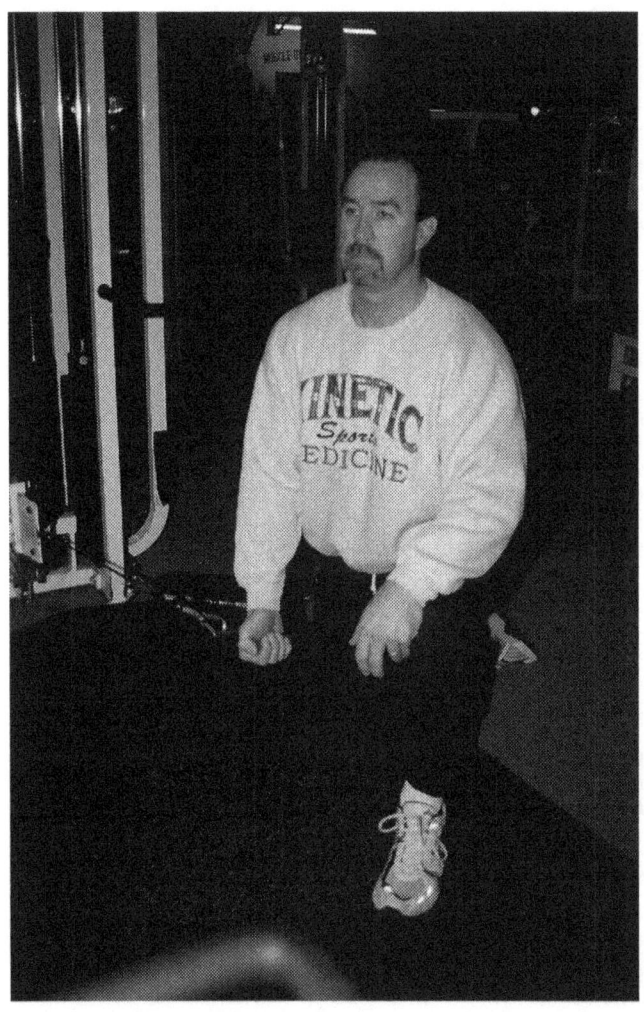

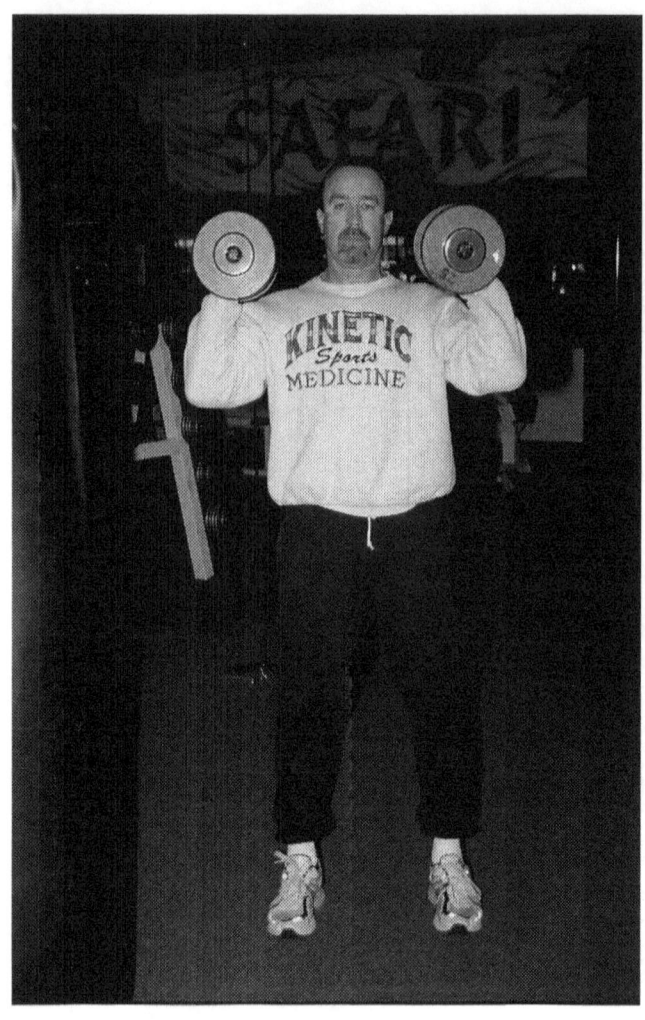

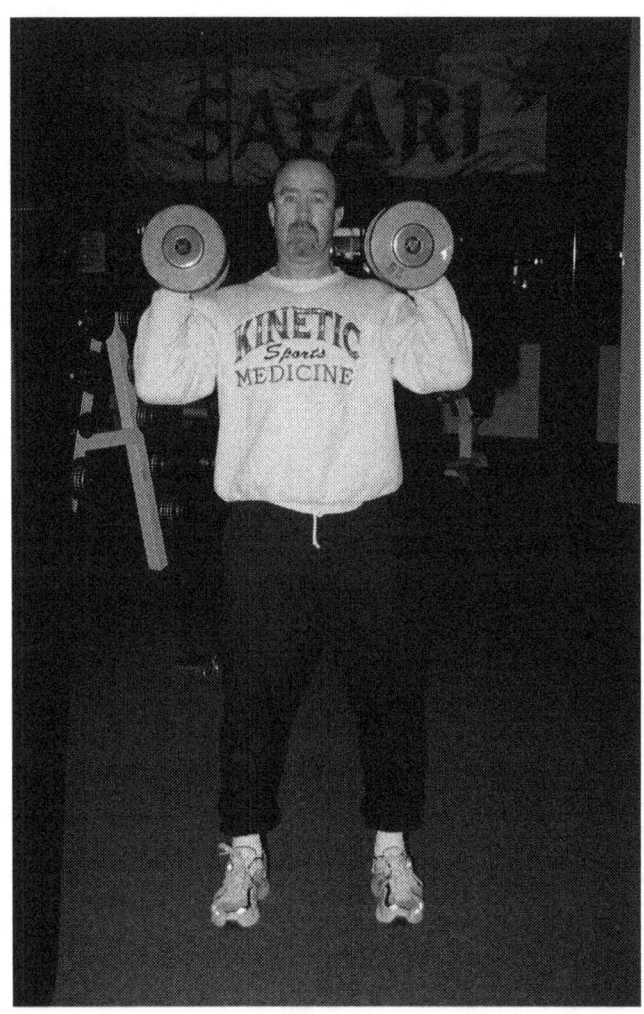

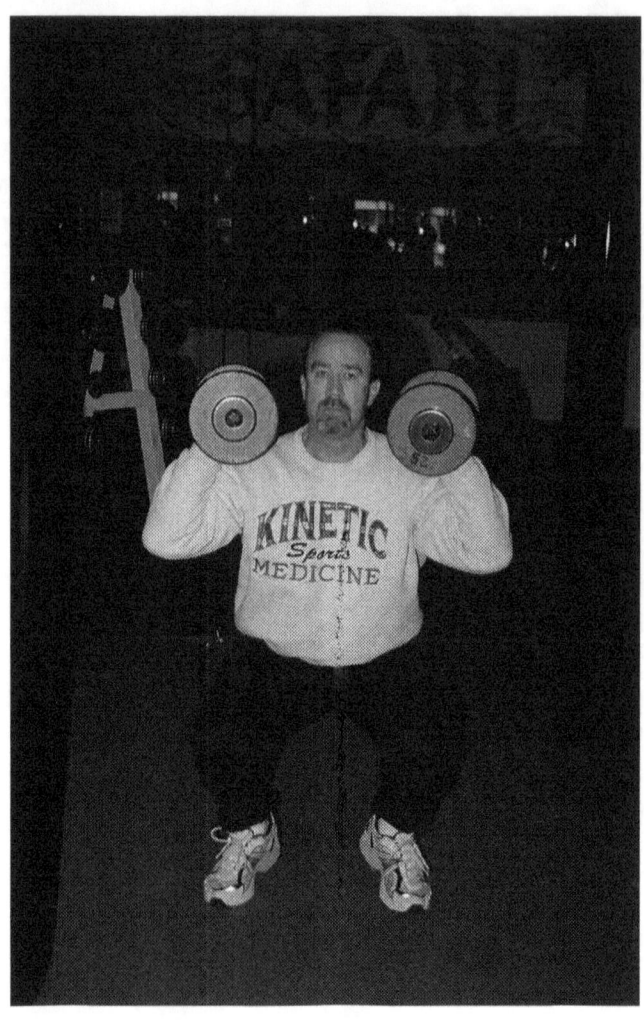

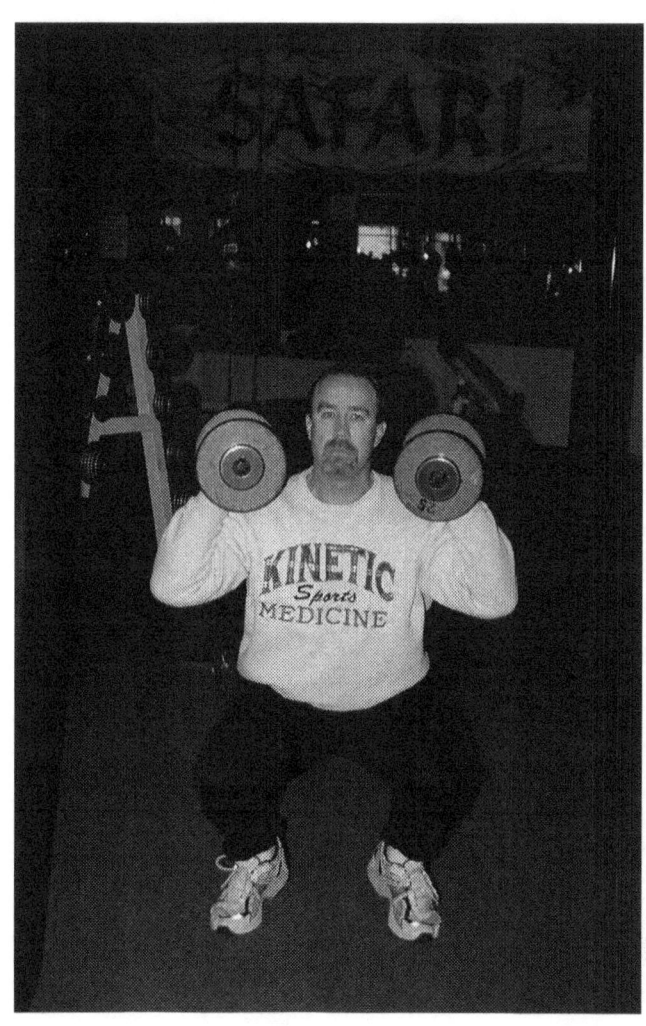

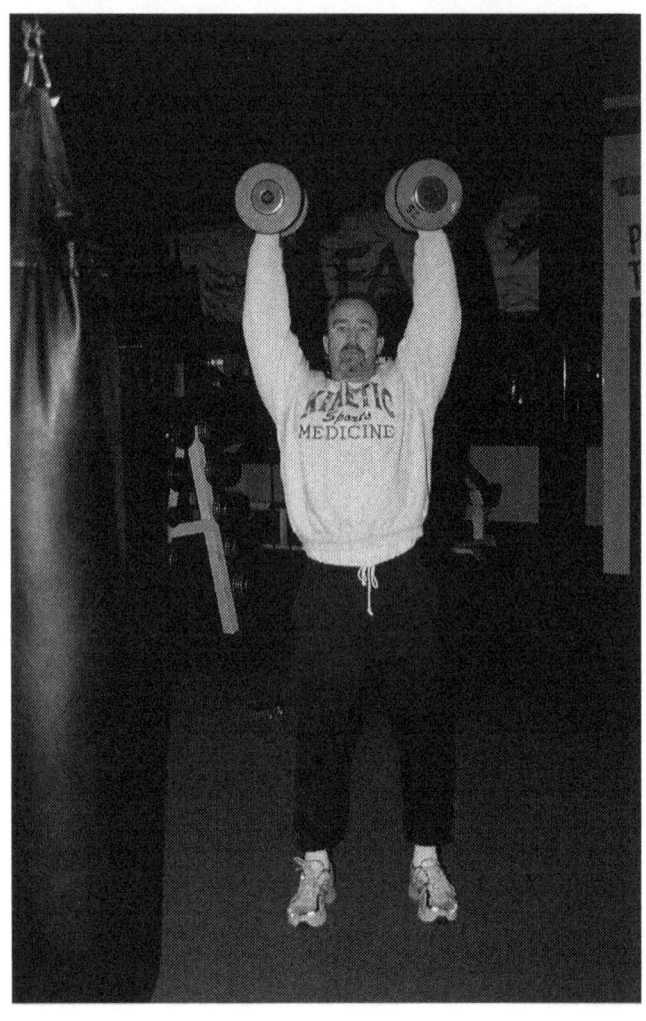

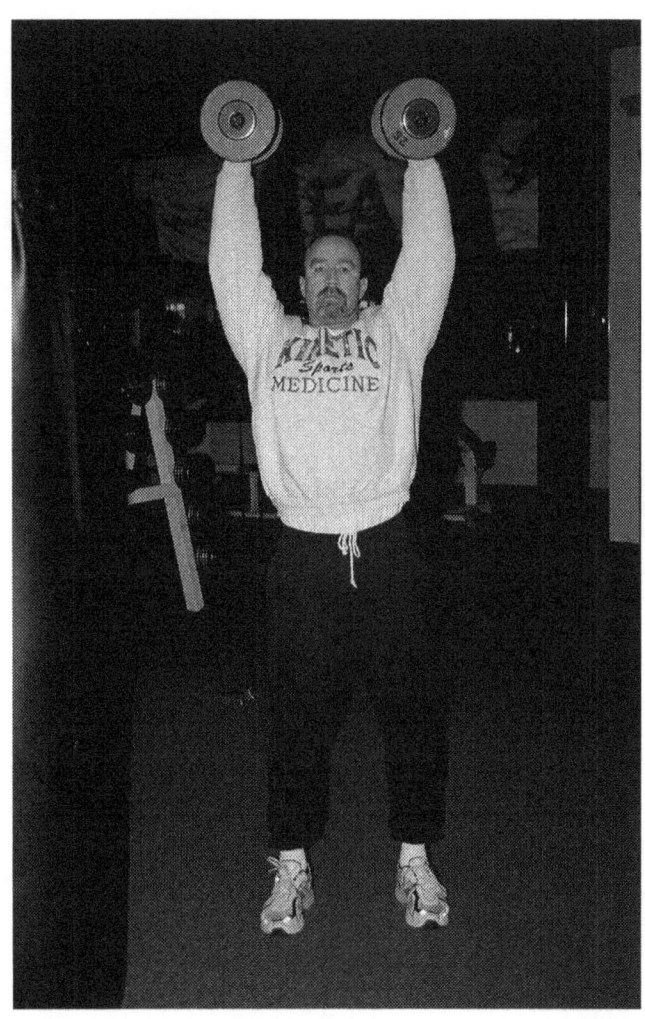

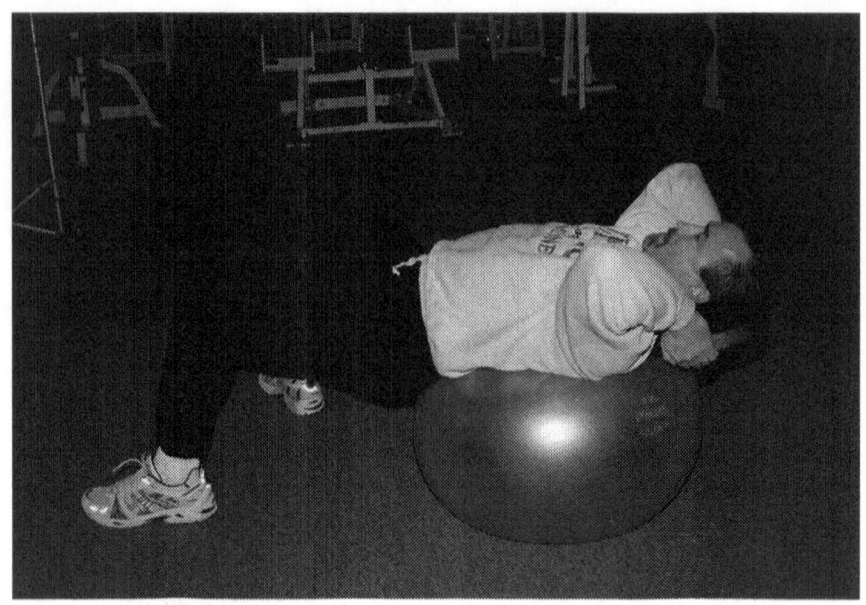

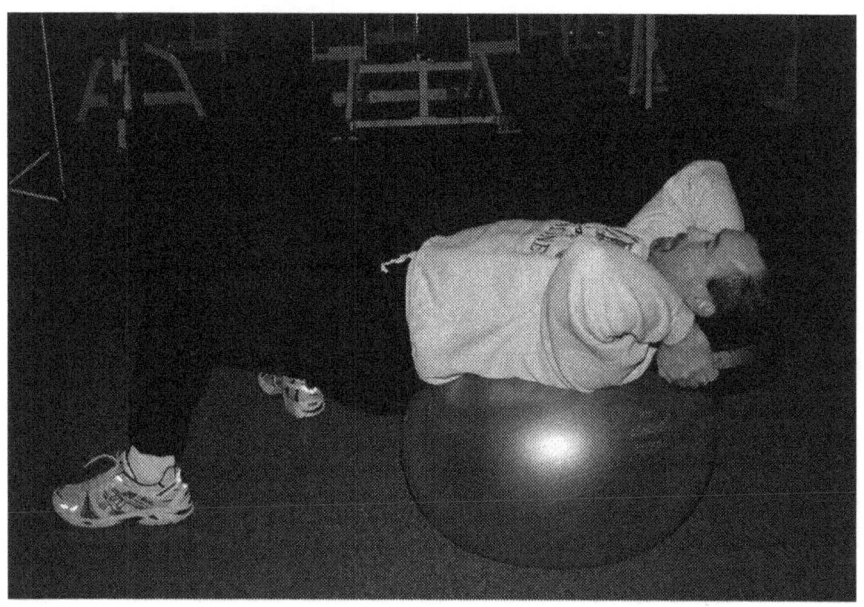

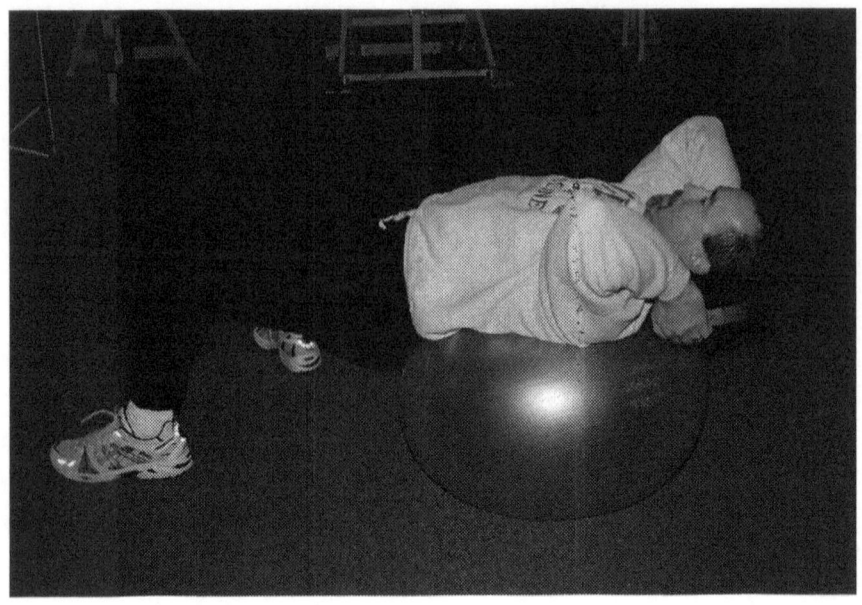

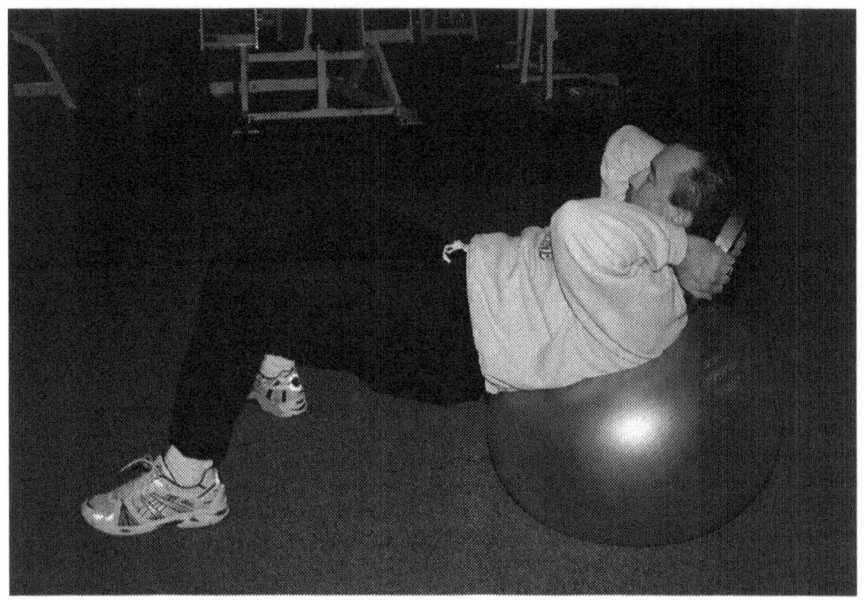

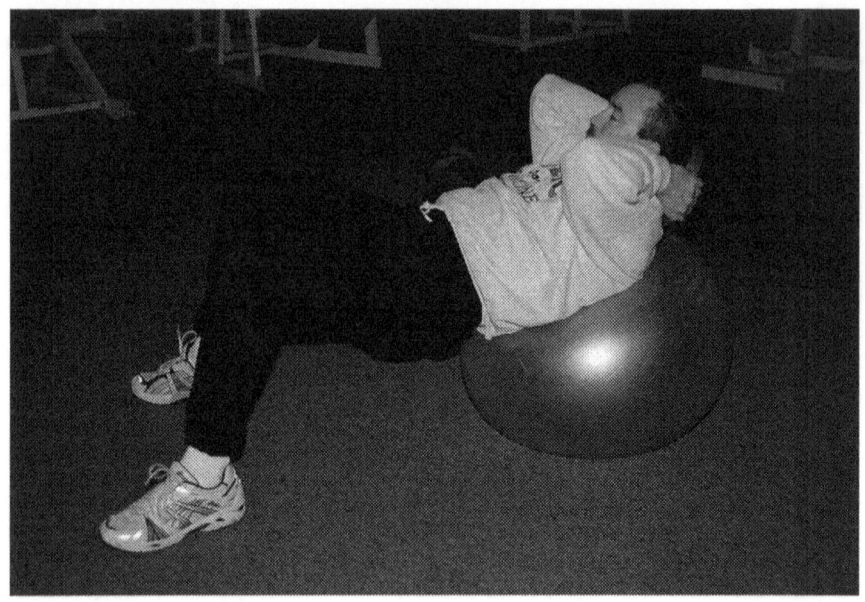

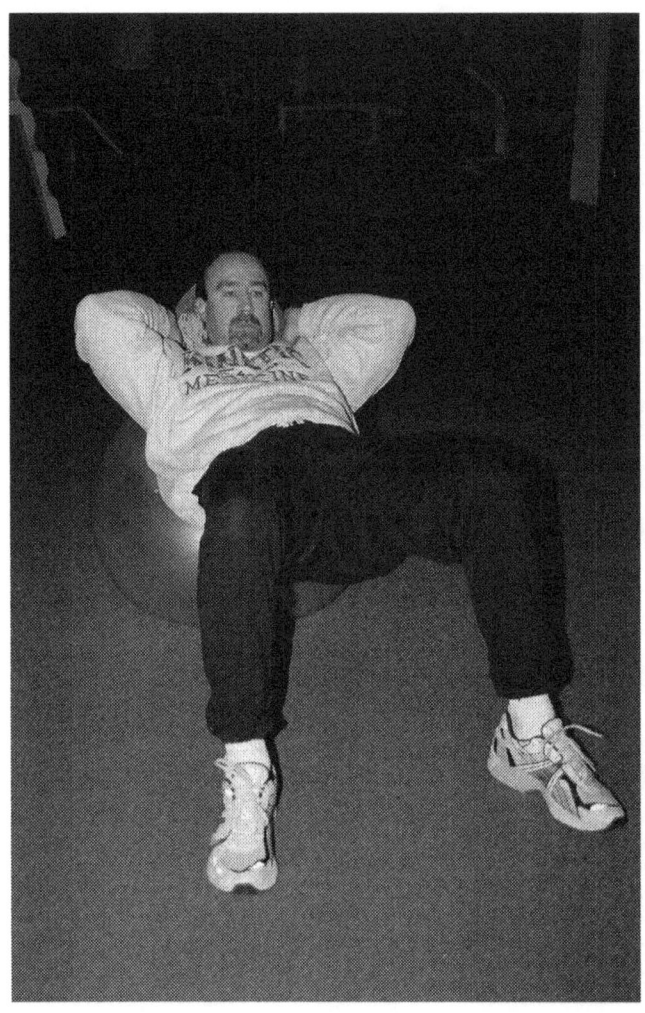

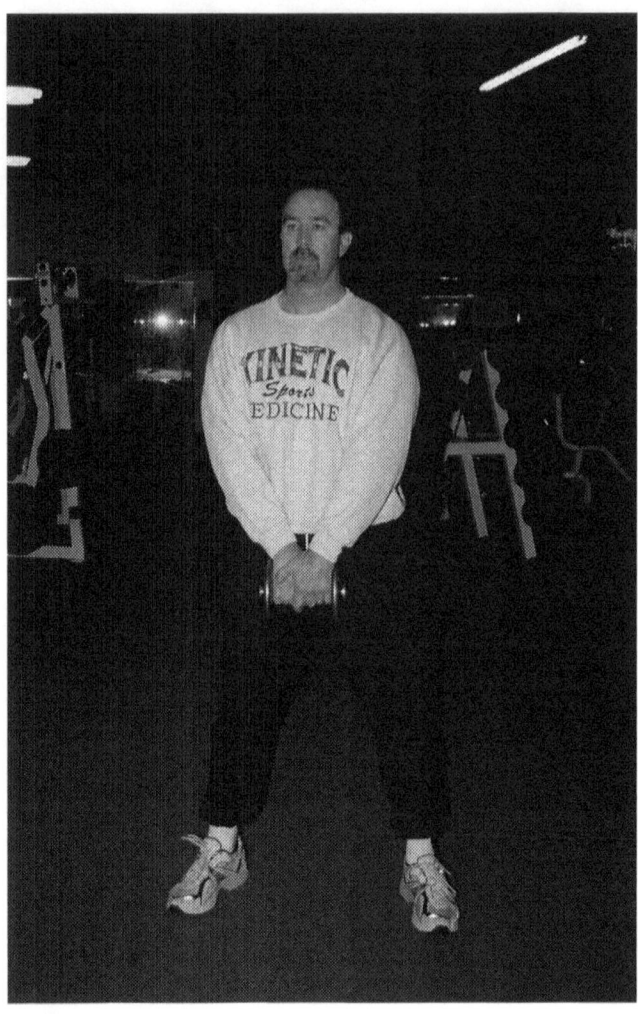

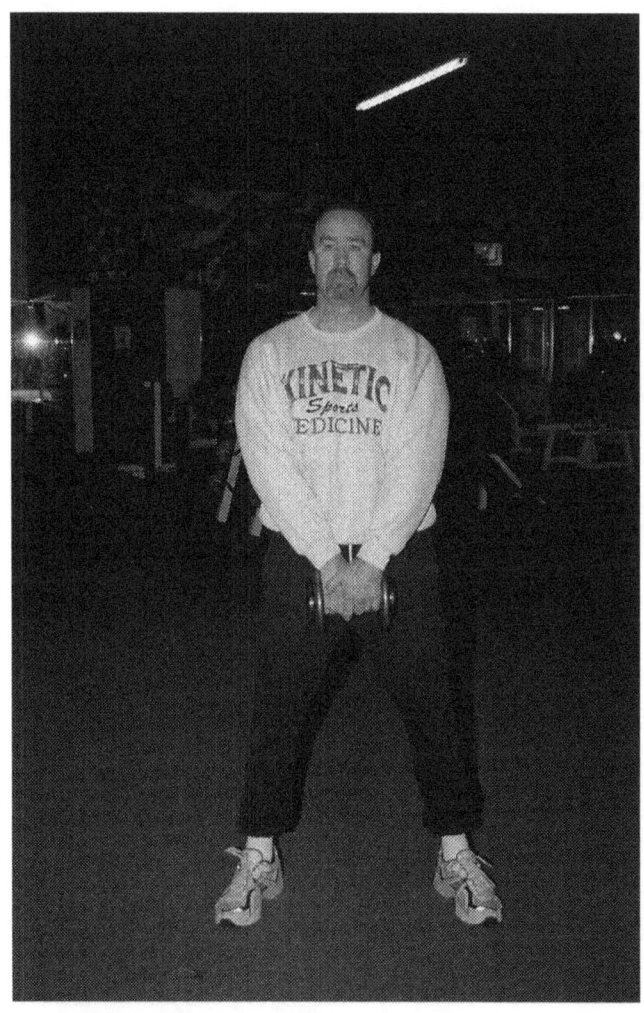

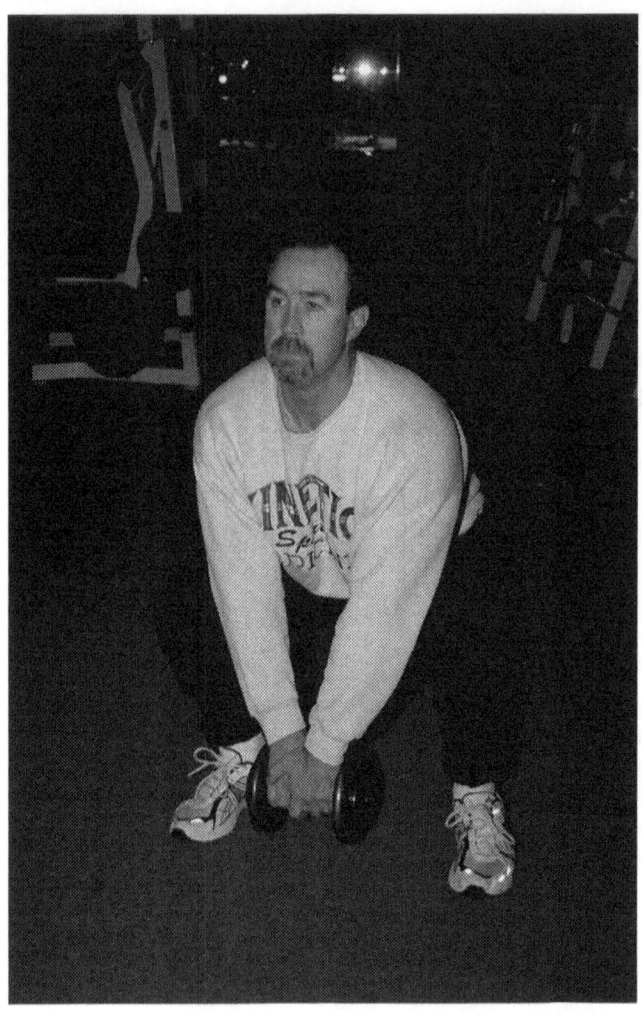

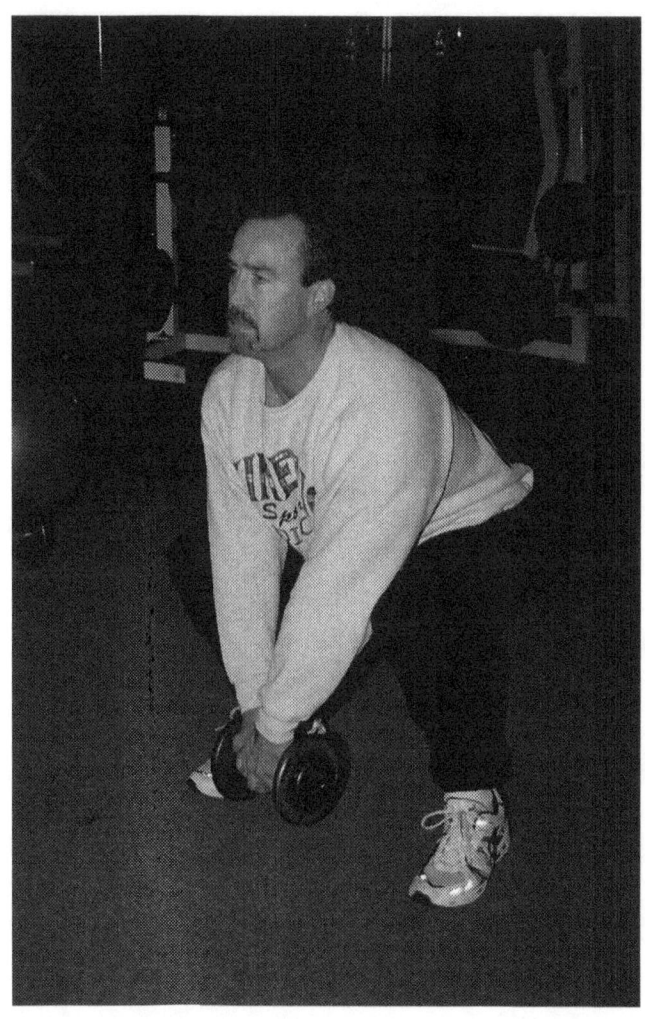

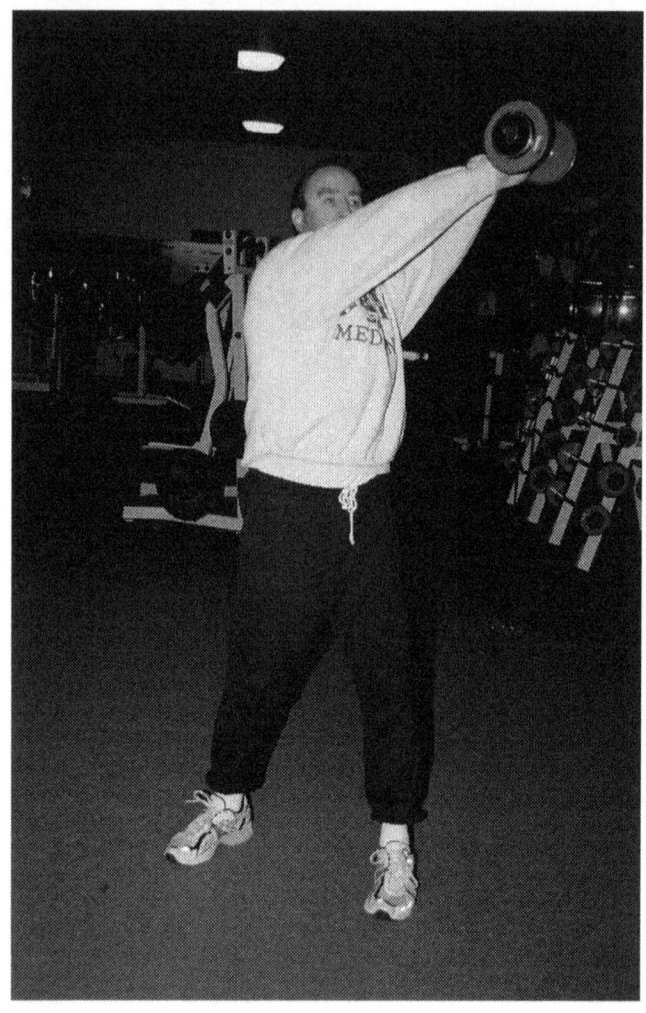

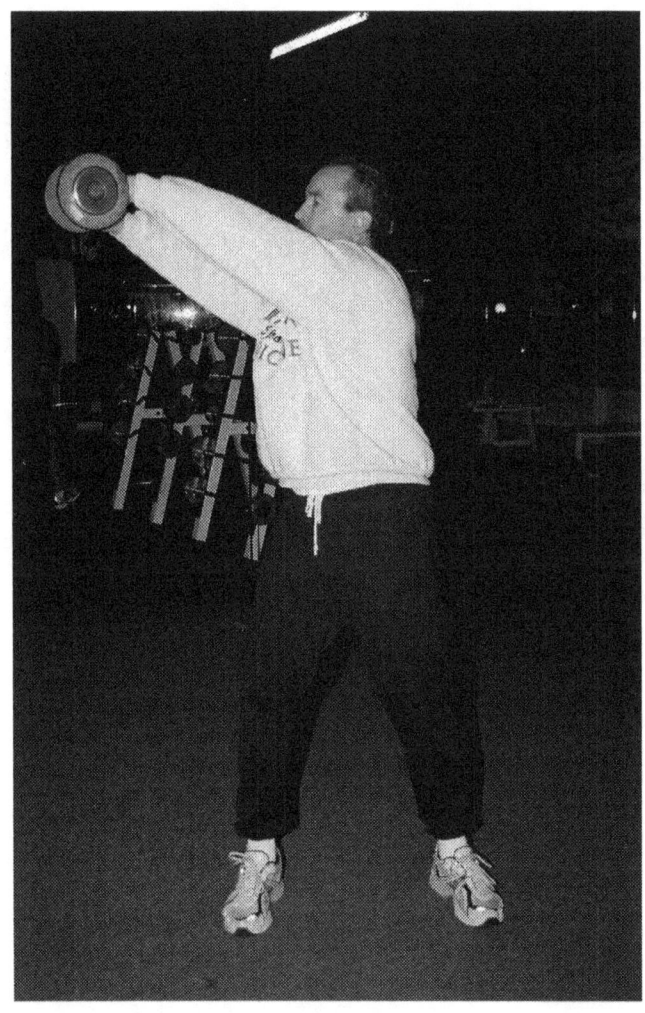

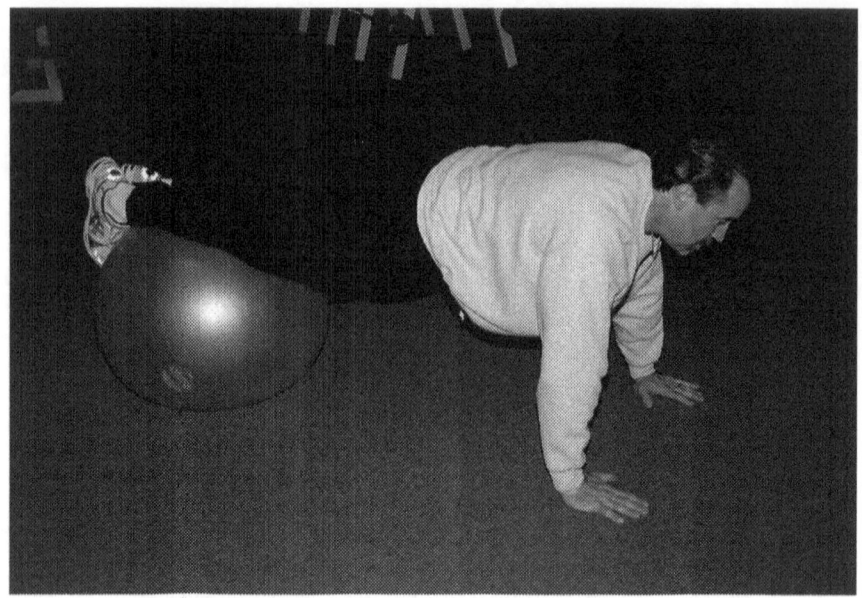

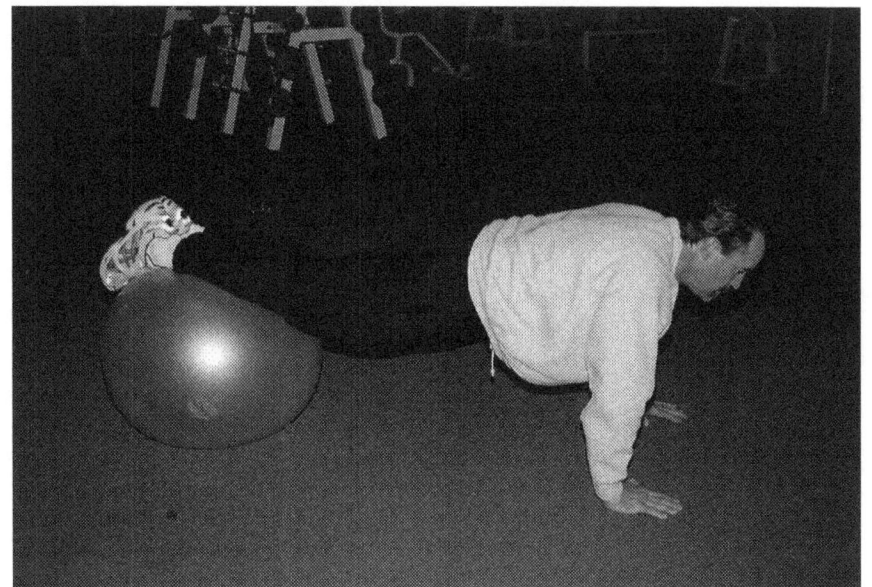

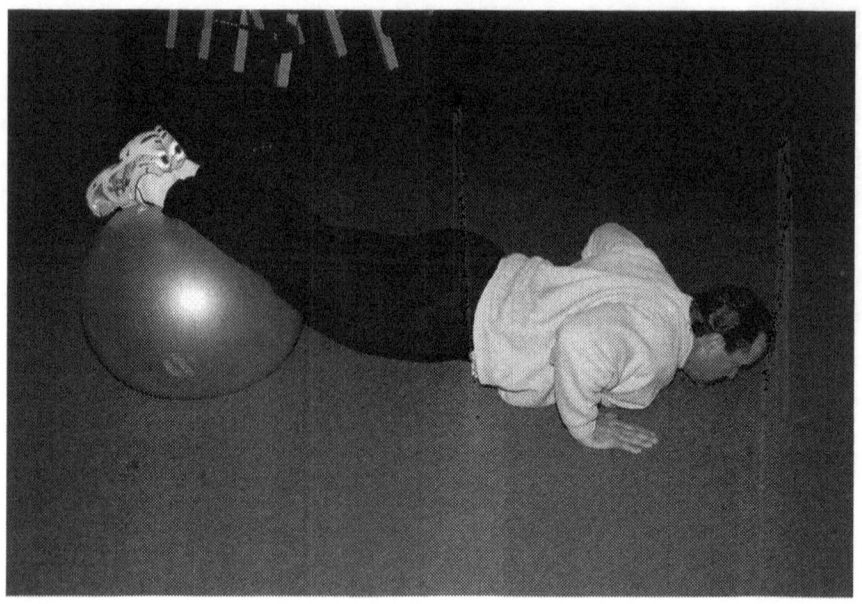

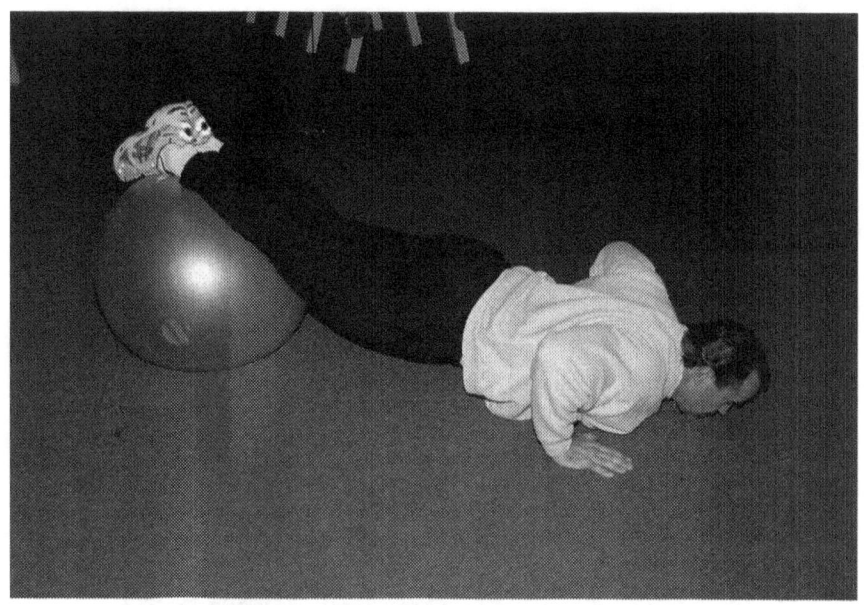

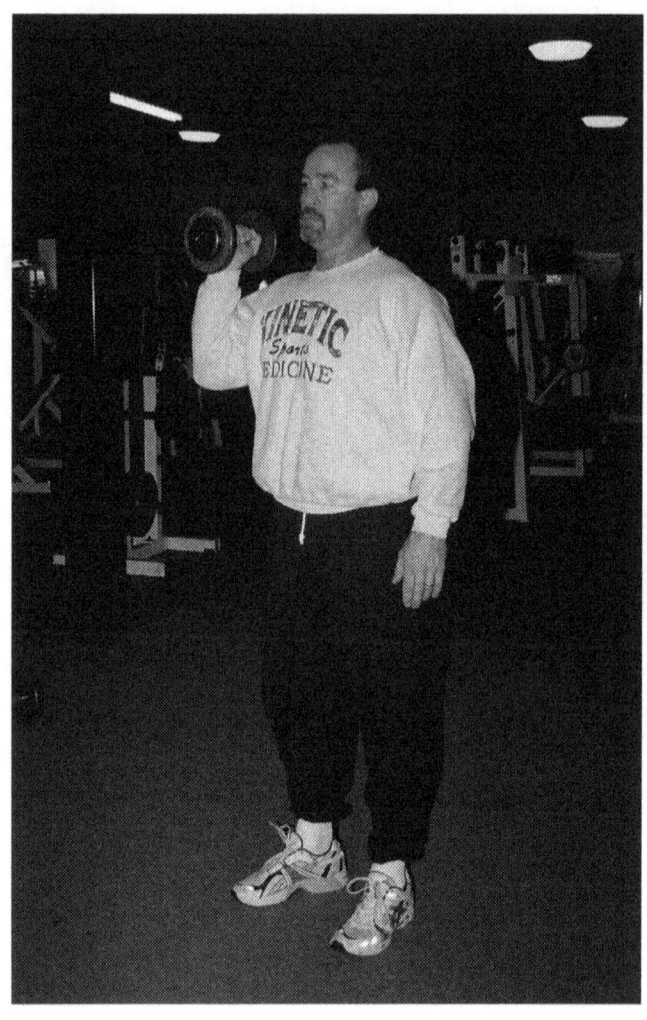

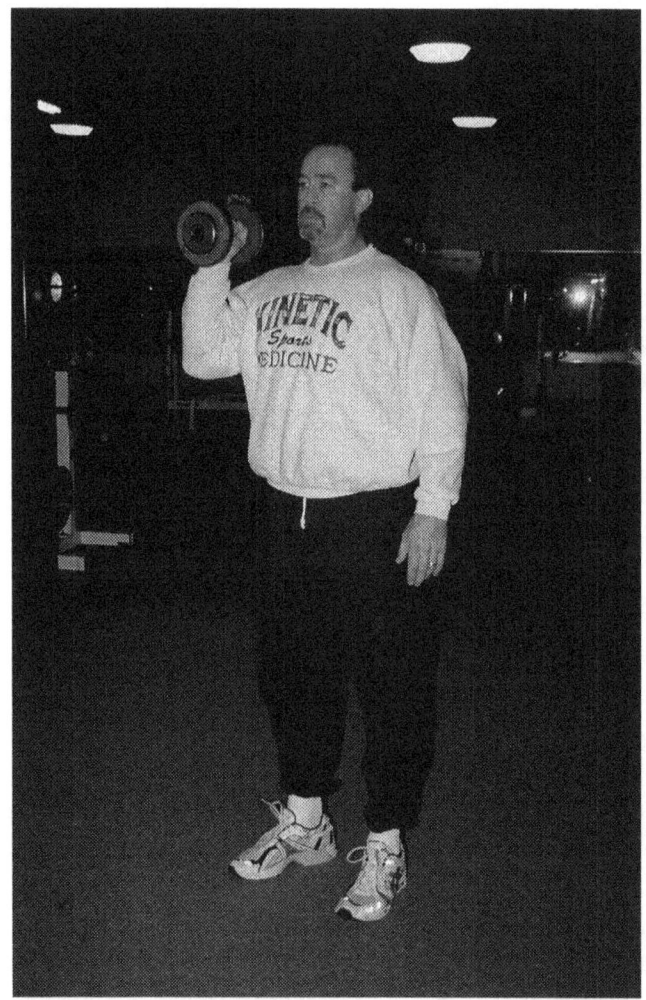

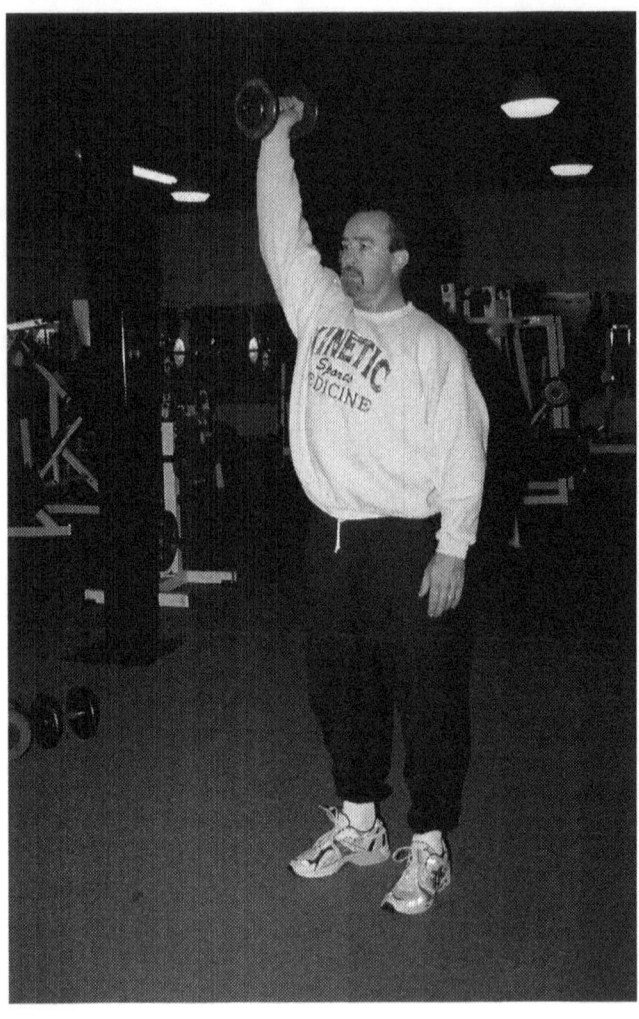

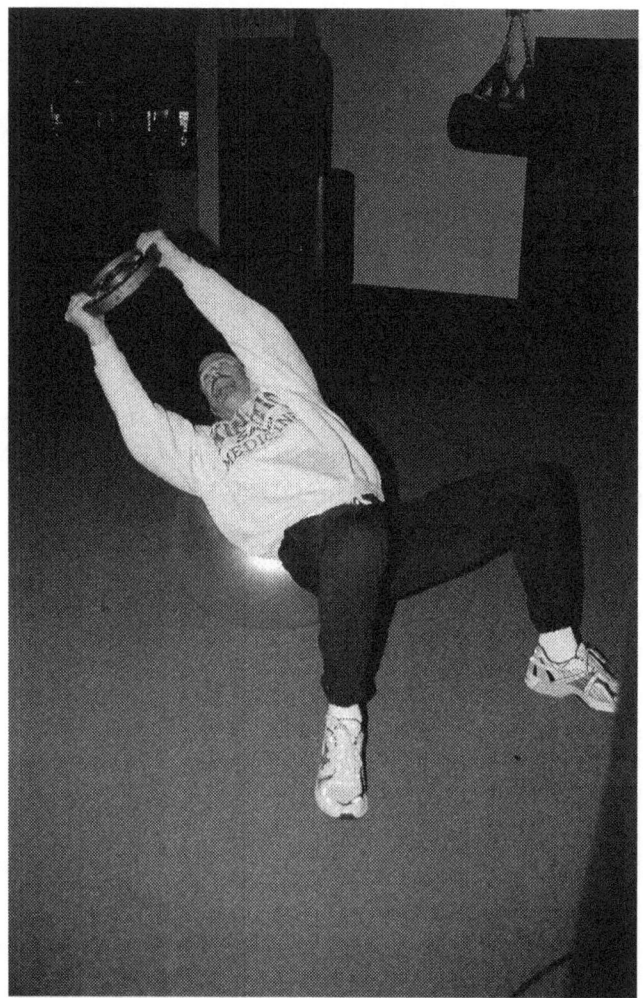

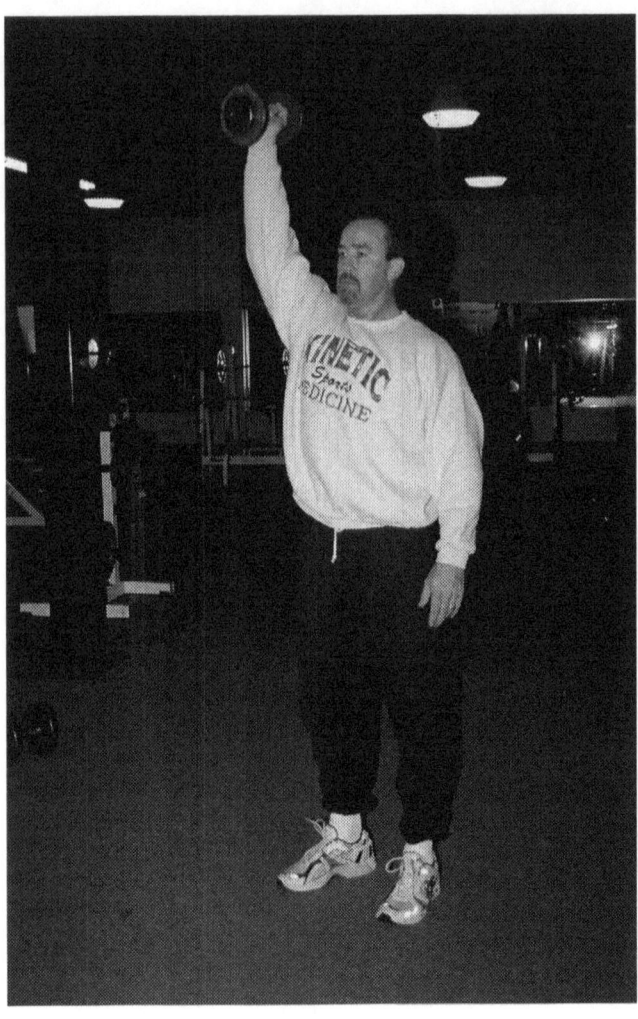

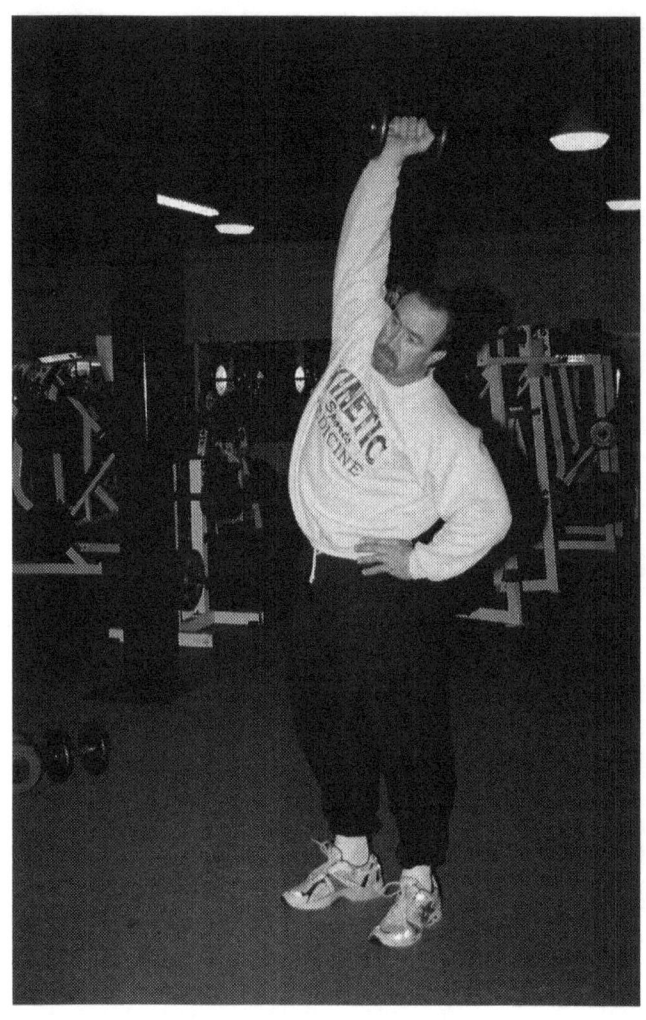

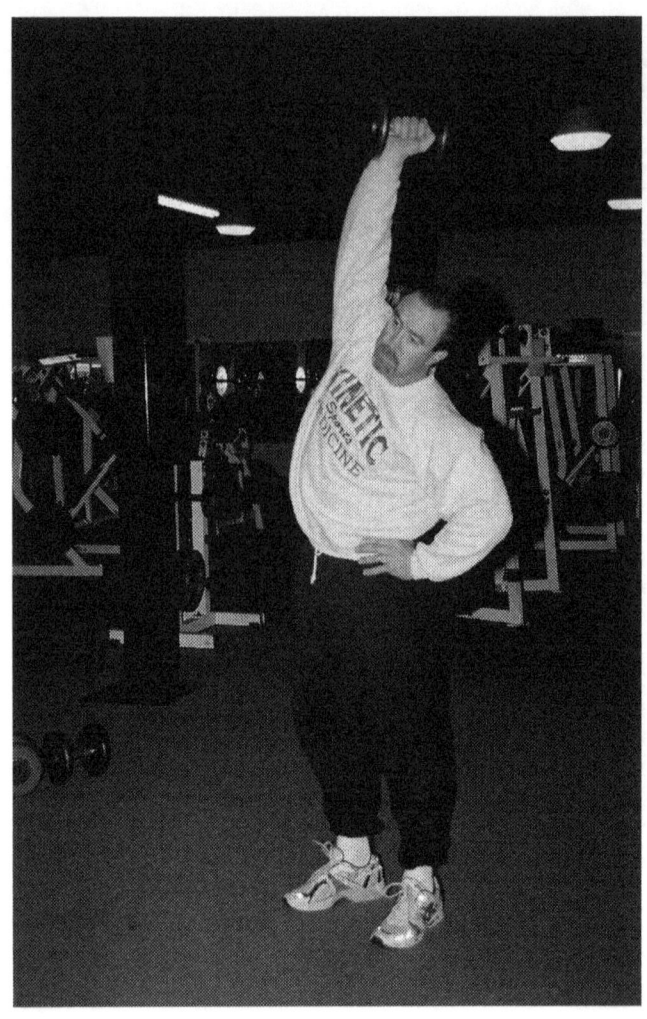

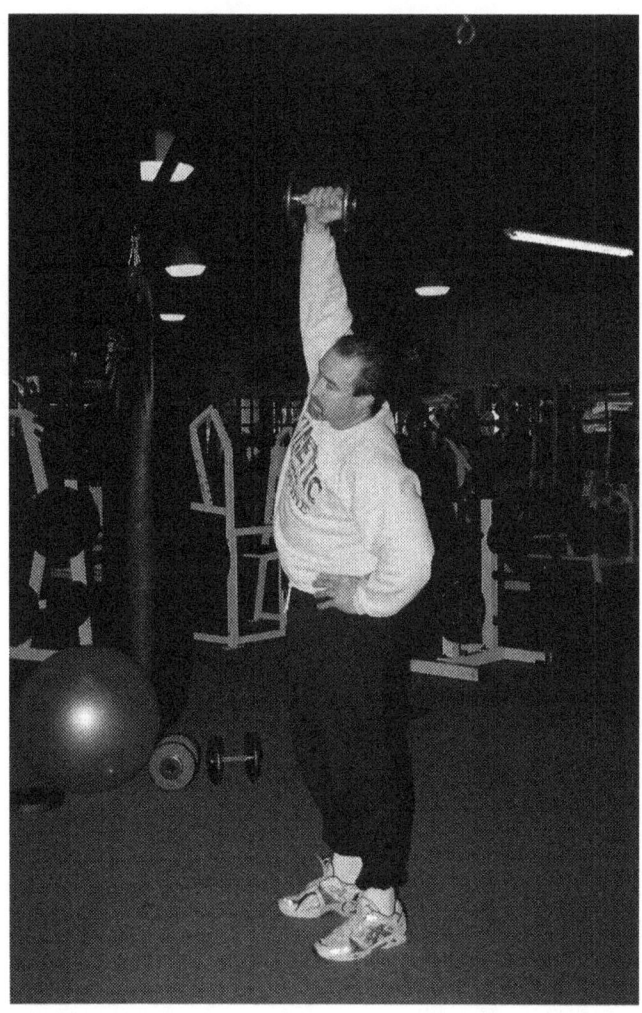

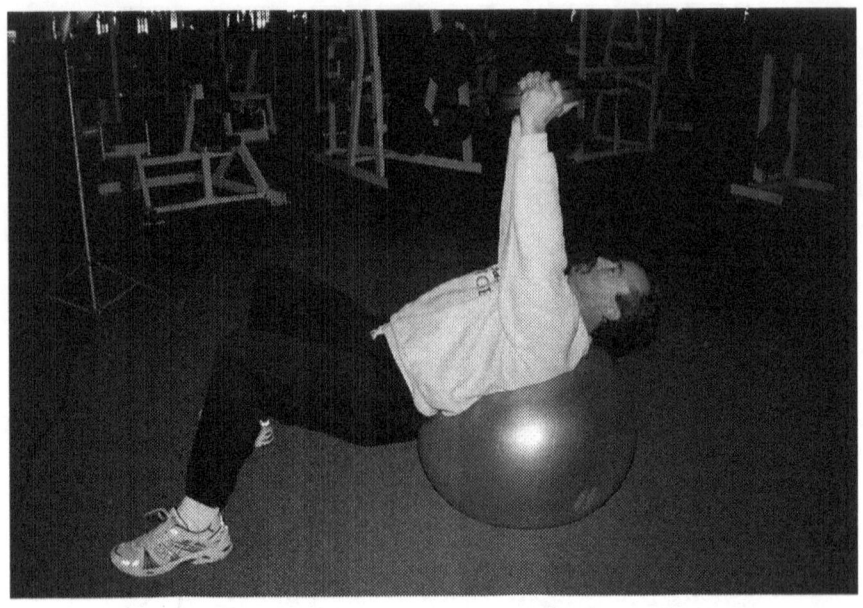

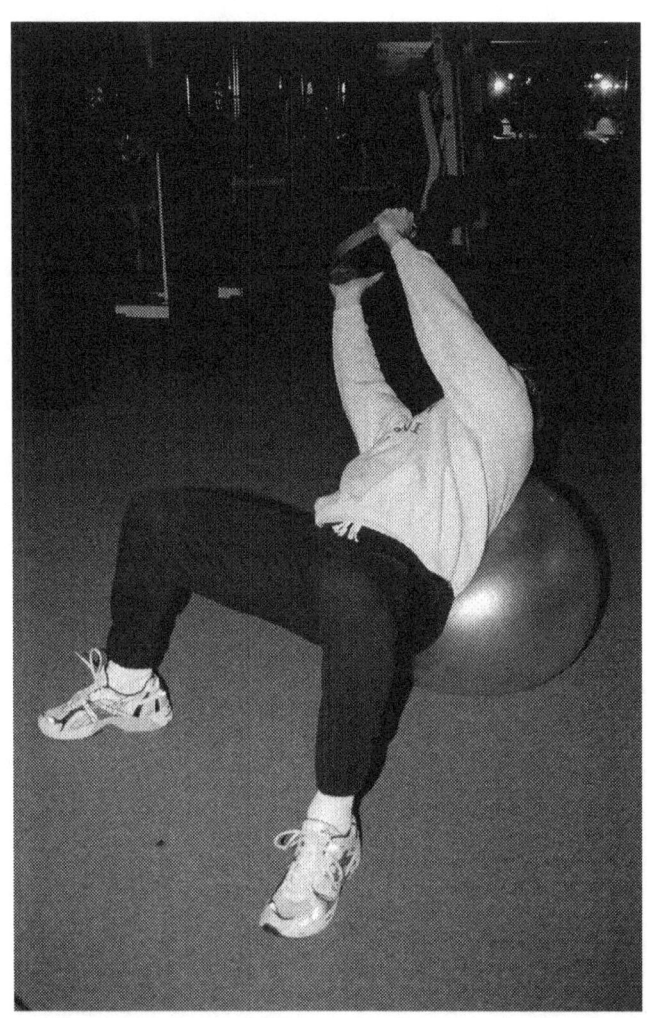

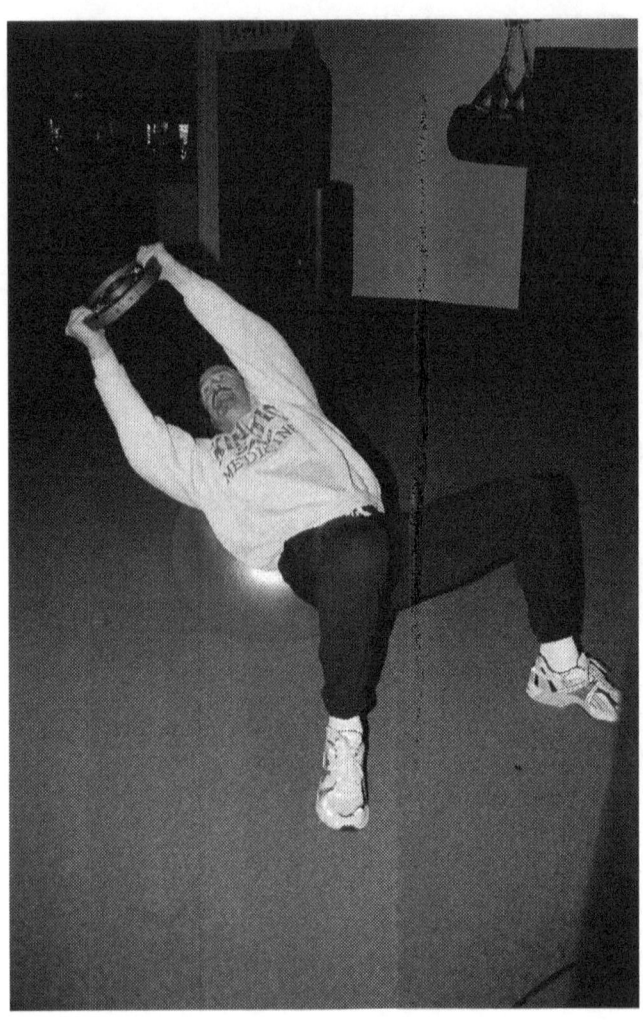

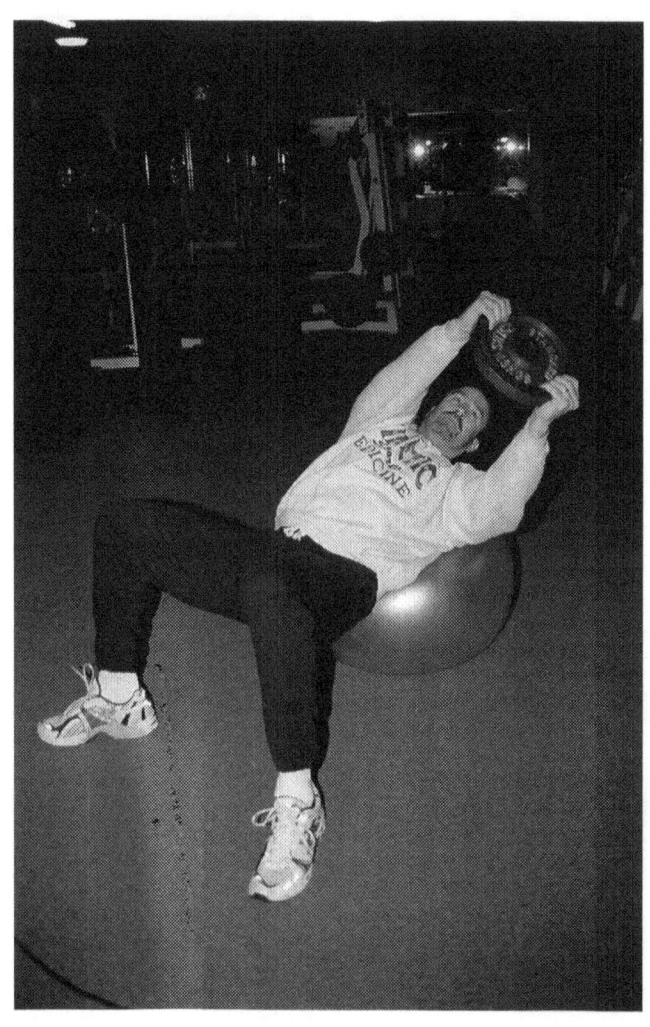

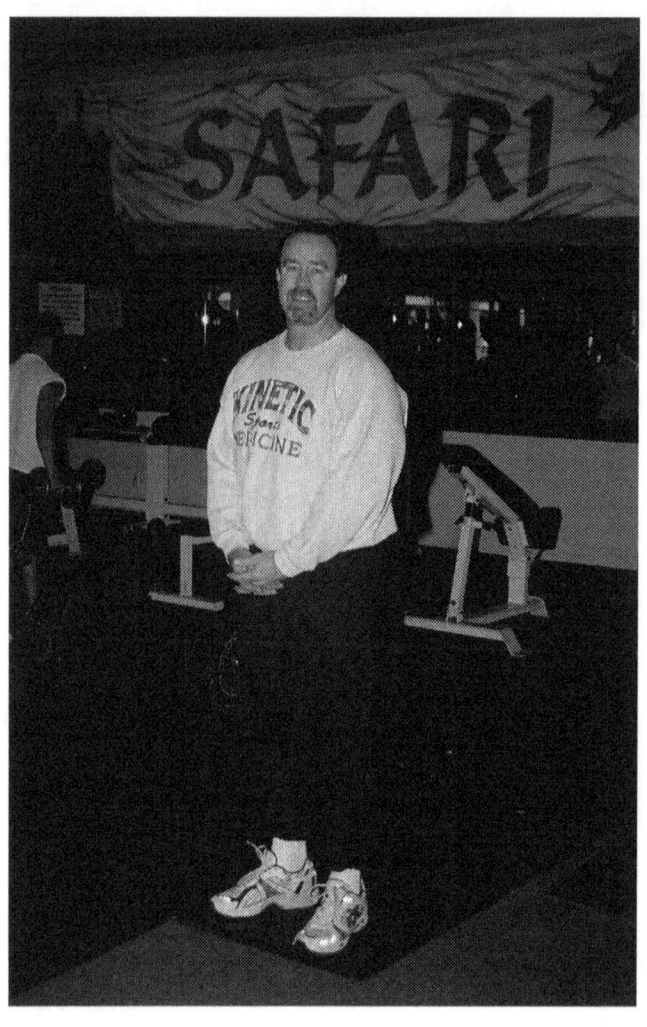

14

Power Walking

✦

For Business Travelers and Ultra-Busy Guys

"Nothing can stop the man with the right mental attitude
From achieving his goal; nothing on earth can help the man
With the wrong mental attitude."

—*Thomas Jefferson*

Guys, this is something you can do anywhere, any time. It's especially great for those of you who travel for your job. You don't have to worry about getting to a gym or if your hotel has a fitness facility. Power walking is easy to do any time! What is *power walking?* It depends on who you ask. Fitness walking is called by many different names—power walking, fitness walking, health walking. Power walking is much more than going out for a stroll. It incorporates the muscles of the upper body making it a *great* aerobic activity. It burns approximately the same calories as a running program, yet it is much easier on the body. Because more muscles are used, power walking will burn calories much quicker than less aggressive walking. It also tones muscles in the buttocks, thighs, hips, shoulders, upper back and abs. Most power walkers cover a mile in about 12 to 15 minutes.

---

40 and Beyond Fitness Tip:

When power walking, don't fall into the mode of "window shopping" and just strolling. Make it count.

See, there's a big difference between fitness walking and mere strolling. Some people fall into the "window shopping" mode when they go for walks simply because the activity is so familiar that it's easy to forget to concentrate on why you are doing it in the first place. But, if you concentrate and do it right, then it can be very beneficial for you. And, the good news is that it doesn't matter what the season is! You can walk any time—any season! It's the easiest, most accessible of fitness activities, requiring no equipment other than a good pair of walking shoes.

So if you're going to use walking or power walking as a way of maintaining fitness levels, there's a few things you should keep in mind to make sure you get the maximum benefit from your sport.

First, find a way to introduce some variety and spice into your walking program. Once adaptation to a certain level of exercise occurs, the body is no longer working very hard to accomplish what once may have taken a lot of effort. Any seasoned exerciser has had some version of this experience: In the beginning, you couldn't do a block without being winded, now a brisk three miler feels like nothing. Or, if you lift weights, at one point, five-pound dumbbells may have felt immovable—now you're doing them for warm-ups.

Unlike race-walking, there is no official definition of power walking. There are no rules. If you walk at a fitness pace three or more miles several times week and cover a mile in 15 minutes or less you are probably power walking.

Use the following tips to insure good walking form and to increase your pace.

Tips for Walking Faster

- Walk tall. Use good posture. Look forward, (not at the ground) gazing about 20 feet ahead. Your chin should be level and your head up.

- Keep your shoulders down, back and relaxed. Chest forward.

- Tighten your abs and buttocks as you walk. Flatten your back and tilt your pelvis slightly forward. Pretend you are walking along a straight line.

- Bend your arms in slightly less than a 90 degree angle. Cup your hands gently. Swing arms front to back (not side to side—arms should not cross your body.) Do not swing elbows higher than your sternum (breastbone). Swing your arms faster and your feet will follow.

- Push off with your toes. Concentrate on striking with the heel, rolling through the step and pushing off with your toes. Use the natural spring of your calf muscles to propel you.

- Resist the urge to elongate your steps. To go faster—take smaller, faster steps.

- Breathe naturally. As you walk, take deep, rhythmic breaths, to get the maximum amount of oxygen through your system.

Walking Don'ts

Here are some common mistakes made by walkers:

- Do not over-stride.

- Do not use too vigorous arm movements.

- Do not look at the ground.

- Do not hunch your shoulders.

- Do not carry hand weights or place weights on your ankles.

Aim for 4 to 6 power walks a week. Beginners should strive to stride for 20 to 30 minutes. More experienced walkers can step it up to 45- or even 60-minute sessions (when time allows). As a rule of thumb, increase your workout time by 10 percent a week. So if you're currently walking 30 minutes a day, 4 days a week, then you should add only 12 minutes to your total weekly walking time the first week you increase. Remember that your workout time includes a few minutes to warm up and a few minutes to cool down and stretch.

40 and Beyond Fitness Tip:

As with any type of exercise, remember to include a few minutes to warm up and a few minutes to cool down and stretch.

Power walking is a great activity that you can do with your girlfriend, friends, wife or children any time, any place. It's the perfect "tool" when you're traveling for business or pleasure. So, men, start walking!

15

Sexy, Yes!

o o o o o o o o o o o o o o o o o o o o o o o o o o o o o o o o o
"The path of freedom does not lead to the goal of freedom:
It is the path of discipline which leads to the goal of liberty."

—*Inayat Khan,* **Notes from the Unstuck Music**

O.K. guys, let's be frank. Men want to feel sexy and stay sexy. We all want to continue to perform like a young buckaroo in the bedroom and when you hit 40, you begin to wonder if your sexual prowess is going to go downhill. It doesn't have to. I promise. And, you don't have to become a subscriber to that little blue pill everyone knows about.

Yep, it's true. The popularity of Viagra has skyrocketed over the past few years. This marvelous little blue pill has brought passion and excitement back into many people's lives. It has proven to be a bestseller with good reason: it's effective for many people. Despite side effects such as headaches and anecdotal reports of possible links to heart attacks, it has helped millions. *But, is it helping them in the long run?*

The problem with a short-term solution such as Viagra, is that it encourages people to forget about seeking treatment. Instead of visiting a doctor to correct the penile dysfunction, most men just pop a pill for instant (thirty minute) results. Viagra is currently the best treatment, but it should be used as a last resort and only after consulting a doctor.

No one can argue that popping a pill is convenient, but penile dysfunction is a complex issue with many causes and manifestations. Even though I am not a doctor and certainly cannot advise people medically, I am using common sense when I say that I caution people against the idea of taking a quick-fix approach to symptoms that are often part of a bigger problem.

40 and Beyond Fitness Tip:

Always consult your physician if you're having problems with penile dysfunction—no matter what your age is!

The first thing you should do before even *thinking* of taking Viagra or any other supplement, is review your overall health and current medications with your doctor. It's also essential to address any psychological or relationship issues through counseling or other forms of therapy. This is very important, because sometimes the problem might be treatable. By taking a quick-fix pop-a-pill approach without investigating the problem, you will only be adding to the delay of treatment and lowering your probability of fully recuperating.

Sure, Viagra is very effective and fast acting—it typically boosts blood flow within 30 minutes to several hours—but some people prefer non-drug alternatives. Is there an alternative to Viagra, something more "natural" like an herb or supplement? And are any of these safe? Not every man requires the magic touch of Viagra; sometimes all one needs is a healthy diet, exercise and a little of Mother Nature's touch. Several interesting supplements have recently come to light and may provide benefits within days to weeks.

Ginkgo Biloba: An herb that is commonly taken as a memory booster may provide benefits. It presumably acts by enhancing blood flow and seems relatively free of side effects. In a study conducted at the University of California, ginkgo reversed sexual problems in 84% of men who were taking antidepressant drugs. The ones who might benefit from it are men on Prozac or other antidepressants. The suggested dose is 80 mg three times a day, standardized to contain 24% flavone glycosides and 6% terpene lactones.

Arginine: An amino acid that also enhances blood flow. In a study of 50 men at Tel Aviv University, 31% of those with impotence improved after six weeks of taking Arginine. The ones who might benefit from it are men who have circulatory disorders that may be contributing to sexual problems. The suggested dose is 1 gram three times a day; sold as L-Arginine.

As with Viagra, you should avoid Arginine if you are taking the heart medication nitroglycerin because the combination may cause a dangerous drop in blood pressure. For the same reason, you should probably not take Arginine with Viagra.

DHEA: This supplement may also provide benefits for men who have low levels of this hormone. DHEA helps our bodies make estrogen and testosterone, and a recent trial at the University of Vienna found it helped men with impotence. The suggested dose is 5 mg each morning for men.

---

40 and Beyond Fitness Tip:

Some studies have shown that the herb, Yohimbe, may correct impotence. Please check with your physician or healthcare practitioner for more information.

Yohimbe: Some studies have shown that this herb may correct impotence. However, this herb can cause a dangerous rise in blood pressure, as well as anxiety and other side effects. Many doctors prefer the purified form of the herb, the FDA-approved drug Yohimbine, instead, because it has a guaranteed purity and potency. I suggest that you opt for the prescription drug Yohimbine instead. See your doctor concerning this.

As for passion potions such as Super Sex and Biagra sold at health-food stores or pharmacies, there is no real evidence showing that they restore sex drive. These potions are made with blends of herbs such as those mentioned above and other questionable ingredients. Check the label to make sure the product contains an adequate dose of the herbs mentioned above. If it does not have the recommended dosages, then the product is not likely to be effective. Instead of a blend, you may be better off purchasing an individual ingredient tailored to your particular condition.

Before taking any of these supplements, please consult your physician or healthcare practitioner. This information is not intended to diagnose or treat, but merely to offer information that has been researched in magazines and books. It is my personal belief that the healthier you are, the sexier you're going to feel! And when you feel sexy, you'll stay sexy no matter what your age!

Little Ways to Feel Sexy

Men, did you know that a great way to feel sexy is to pay attention to what women want and embrace things that make *them* feel sexy. Following are some examples of what you can do to put romance back into your life (if it's missing) and to feel sexy while doing it!

- Go for a walk in the rain on a warm summer day with your loved one, hand-in-hand. Let the water soak through your shirt. *She* will make you feel sexier than you've ever felt before!

- Write your wife or girlfriend a lusty passionate letter. Begin by telling her all the things you find so sexy about her: her long legs, the way her eyes crinkle when she smiles, the sound she makes when you touch her. Then describe all the *hot* things you plan on doing to her tonight. Putting your frisky feelings into words will seriously fire up your desire and make you and your significant other *feel* alive and sexy.

- Be submissive for once. If you've fallen into the role of being bossy and authoritative when it comes to initiating some action, be a little passive and let her take the lead. She will love feeling powerful and will make you feel very, *very* desirable!

- Inch into her personal space. You'll create an electric buzz between the two of you. Just hold your conversation about a foot closer than you normally would and stare into her eyes. You'll soon find that you can't finish your sentences, because you're both so focused on that surging sexual energy.

- Flirt with your lady. Honestly, when was the last time you really doted on your woman? Forever ago? Well, pretend she's a new girlfriend—a new date—and chuckle at her jokes, suggestively touch her forearm and make coy comments. You'll feel the excitement of a first date—a first kiss—all over again.

- Wear leather. A leather jacket with blue jeans is just the thing to make you feel sexy. Women love leather. There's just something so masculine and sexy about it for *women!*

- Forget a towel when you take a shower, then call to your lady to bring you one. When she enters the steamy room, let her see your totally soaped-up body. Invite her to join you. *When was the last time you did that?* Water is an aphrodisiac and she'll be more than happy to succumb. Then, wash her hair for her. If you remember the scene in *Out of Africa* where Robert Redford washes Meryl Streep's hair, you'll understand what I mean. There's nothing quite so sexy as when you wash a woman's hair. The soft, sexy way she feels will make *you* feel sexier than you've ever felt before.

- Describe steamy dreams—about *her*, of course—*not* the one about you and Pamela Anderson! Spare no detail, such as how your skin felt, where she touched you, where the tryst took place. Just reliving the fantasy will get you hot and bothered, and she'll be inspired to make it come true.

- Give your wife or girlfriend a sexy invite. Slip a penny or a little horseshoe charm in her purse with a note that says, "You're getting lucky tonight." All day you'll both be percolating with sexy thoughts of the very exciting evening ahead.

- Whenever you're having a cocktail in a bar, order yourself a piña colada with two straws. That pineapple-coconut combo just oozes sexiness and women love these kinds of drinks. Think about it: You never associate this tantalizing cocktail with anything but soft sand, warm sun rays and semi-nakedness. Let the tropical scent transport you to a racy mental place.

- Put away your PJs, your sweats, your boxer shorts. We spend most of our lives dressed, so sleeping nude will remind you of just how sensual and sexy you can feel in your skin. And, you won't hear her complaining. Nothing makes a guy feel sexier than sleeping in the nude.

The best thing you can do though to really feel sexy about yourself is to eat right, exercise, and be as healthy as you can. That is where real sexiness comes from.

16

Stayin' the Course

"You may be disappointed if you fail, but you are doomed if you don't try."

—*Beverly Sills*

Many so-called experts predict that our aging generation will become an albatross around America's neck—overwhelming the health care system, bankrupting Social Security, hoarding our wealth, and retreating to retirement villages where we'll refuse to support schools and social services with our taxes. I don't think this is necessarily the case.

Life After 40 Can Be Your Best Years Yet!

That's right, guys. We are a generation of revolution and new ideas. We're changing everything we've ever cared about, from how we raise our kids to how we relate in the workplace. Now we care about aging, and we're going to do it like it's never been done before! By utilizing the simple steps I've outlined in this book, being older can mean being healthier, wiser, and sexier than ever.

If you believe that getting older means struggling to live within your means, falling apart at the seams, and giving up on your dreams, then perhaps you haven't enjoyed this book. But if you want to make life after 40 your *best* years yet—if you're looking for new ideas, new concepts, and new adventures—then get ready to rock and roll! Hopefully, now that you've read this book, you'll agree that you now look at aging altogether differently.

Unlike the previous generations, whose memories of the Great Depression and World War II left them worried about the future and world events, we have always been creative, optimistic, unafraid of change, and young at heart. We believe the best is yet to come. Or, at least that's how we should believe. Guys, you've simply got to realize that being 40 is not old. It is the beginning of the rest of your life!

I don't plan to ever consider myself a "senior," no matter how old I get. I am living a lifestyle I love and I don't want it to end. Rather than retiring to inactivity, I feel like a kid out of high school and in life I have a number of options. This is the way to stay young—by realizing that the world is waiting for you to embrace it. If you want to stop one career, then you have a number of options before you. Many opportunities are ours for the taking, and with a little planning, we'll have the wisdom, insight, intuition, and money to make our dreams come true.

We "over 40" guys are a generation of revolution and new ideas. We've changed everything we've ever cared about and now we care about aging, and we're going to do it like it's never been done before.

---

40 and Beyond Fitness Tip:

We "over 40" guys are a generation of revolution and new ideas.

Life after 40 can be our best years yet, but a life of health and total abundance won't happen automatically. To enjoy healthy longevity, we'll have to create the possibility for it to occur. You'll need to develop the physical, mental, spiritual, emotional—and yes, financial—readiness to face what many consider the retirement years. Since we're likely to live longer than we may have imagined, we may need or want to continue working beyond age 65. To do that, we'll need to be in good shape physically, financially, mentally, and emotionally.

I hope that my book has helped you and that you're embracing all the keys to exercise, nutrition, and health care that I've outlined for you. Taking advantage of all the opportunities available to you—fitness centers, health clubs, sports, numerous nutritional food plans—plus continuing to work or starting a new career, traveling, mentoring the younger generation, and enjoying the things you're passionate about—will be much more fun and enjoyable if you're in the best physical condition you can possibly achieve.

What do we guys have to look forward to? We have a simple choice: We can define your future life or let others define it for us. I for one, intend to be a definer, not a definee. I've already begun envisioning my future, and so can you. You can stay the course by using this book as a guide. Keep it in your briefcase or in your desk drawer at work. Refer to it any time you start to feel old and remember, *you're not old!*

By the way, you don't have to be over 40 to benefit from this book. If you want to be sure you'll have the health and energy to live the way you want and contribute to your family and community in meaningful ways, it's never too soon to start planning your future. A *healthier, younger, sexier* future.

That future can start now, today. Are you ready?

About the Author

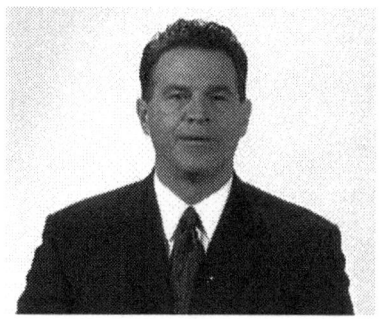

For more than 20 years, Tony Vercillo has been sharing his secrets to success and good health with audiences around the world. A gifted and dynamic public presenter, Vercillo has been a featured keynote speaker at international conferences, seminars and corporate meetings. One of America's leading consultants, entrepreneurs, and health-care enthusiasts, Vercillo had a wake-up call on his 40th birthday and decided to change his life.

Tony splits his time between Las Vegas and Southern California where he coaches youth sports and teaches at a local university.

0-595-33910-7

www.ingramcontent.com/pod-product-compliance
Lightning Source LLC
Chambersburg PA
CBHW061257280526
45784CB00002B/797